The International Library of Psychology

THOUGHT AND THE BRAIN

Founded by C. K. Ogden

The International Library of Psychology

PHYSIOLOGICAL PSYCHOLOGY
In 10 Volumes

I	Pleasure and Instinct	*Allen*
II	Pleasure and Pain	*Bousfield*
III	The Neural Basis of Thought	*Campion et al*
IV	Body and Mature Behaviour	*Feldenkrais*
V	Emotions of Normal People	*Marston et al*
VI	Integrative Psychology	*Marston et al*
VII	The Development of the Sexual Impulses	*Money-Kyrle*
VIII	The Laws of Feeling	*Paulhan*
IX	Thought and the Brain	*Piéron*
X	The Image and Appearance of the Human Body	*Schilder*

THOUGHT AND THE BRAIN

HENRI PIÉRON

Routledge
Taylor & Francis Group
LONDON AND NEW YORK

First published in 1927 by
Routledge, Trench, Trubner & Co., Ltd.
2 Park Square, Milton Park, Abingdon, Oxfordshire OX14 4RN
711 Third Avenue, New York, NY 10017

First issued in paperback 2014

Routledge is an imprint of the Taylor and Francis Group, an informa business

British Library Cataloguing in Publication Data
A CIP catalogue record for this book
is available from the British Library

Thought and the Brain
ISBN 0415-21080-1
Physiological Psychology: 10 Volumes
ISBN 0415-21131-X
The International Library of Psychology: 204 Volumes
ISBN 0415-19132-7

ISBN 13: 978-1-138-87551-7 (pbk)
ISBN 13: 978-0-415-21080-5 (hbk)

CONTENTS

CHAPTER III

PART II

THE RECEPTIVE AND INCITO-MOTOR FUNCTIONS

(The elementary modes of sensori-motor thought).

PREFACE

In any attempt to solve the problem of human thought, it is not easy to avoid the influence of preconceptions and the tendency to accept certain assumptions with undue indulgence while rejecting others with excessive severity.

Without prejudice in favour of any particular theory, the author has confined himself to the examination of various questions which he does not by any means claim to have solved, but which he considers are capable of being stated with some degree of precision in view of the scientific knowledge now at our disposal.

The ideal of science is the highest possible degree of unification, and it undoubtedly aims at the correlation of psychological facts with physiological mechanics, neglecting the subjective aspect of consciousness. This effort to attain unity, which, according to the profound views of Emile Meyerson, responds to the fundamental craving after unity inherent in the human mind, has an undeniable value in research. Whatever certain theorists may assert to the contrary, neurophysiology does undoubtedly often provide an adequate representation of the laws established by psychology, as will be seen in the course of the present work; the study of the functions of the brain frequently supplies a satisfactory explanation of psychological phenomena. In fact, we often pass from one form of representation—or rather, from one form of expression or language—to the other.

To these and similar advances made by science, beliefs will always adapt themselves. If it is a materialistic doctrine that seeks support from the new data, the adaptation presents no difficulty. But even a spiritualistic creed, if free to remould certain articles of faith, could well accept the facts now established. There will always be a sufficient residue of the unknown for scientific facts to be accommodated to the various systems of beliefs; and in any case the mind can always take refuge in a transcendental idealism.

Moreover, the identification of the physiological with the mental can be readily admitted by an animistic vitalism which requires some underlying spiritual principle—a Life-Force, or something similar—as an explanation of life in all its manifestations. Metaphysical theory, however, is of small account in the single quest for scientific truth; for this is the only possible basis of agreement among genuine inquirers; and by its means alone can our collective inheritance be enriched. It might, indeed, be claimed as the only 'truth,' but that would be a gratuitous introduction of a new form of faith.

H. P.

THOUGHT AND THE BRAIN

PART I

THE GENERAL CONCEPTION OF NEURO-MENTAL FUNCTIONING

INTRODUCTION

SOME years ago our conception of cerebral mechanisms and of the functioning of the nervous system in general passed through an evolutionary crisis. Then came the War, and the countless nervous lesions for which it was responsible, constituting a real physio-pathological experiment on a huge scale, with results whose inventory is not complete even to-day. No mean body of knowledge is now at our disposal as to the functioning of the human nervous system. In particular, everything that concerns the reflex organization, the rôle of the sympathetic system or of the nervous conductors, is very much better understood. But at first sight the same does not seem to be true of the cerebral functions, since contradictions appear to emerge from the facts ascertained. On the one hand there is the view that cerebral localization can be determined and completed by the examination of strictly limited lesions, involving well-defined partial defects; while on the other hand the fact that there are general disturbances which, whatever the lesion, remain the same, and the absence of serious disturbances in spite of very considerable lesions, have once more cast doubts on the theory of localization.

Before examining more closely the data which have given rise to such contradictory tendencies, it is necessary both to recall what the brain represents from the standpoint of comparative physiology, and also to ascertain the main lines on which this organ functions from the standpoint of psycho-physiology.

Very erroneous ideas are certainly still prevalent in these branches of science, especially as regards psycho-physiology among those who study the brain, and as regards 'cerebrology' among those who are concerned with psychological analysis. And to these false ideas are due the disagreement and contradiction on questions relating to cerebral function which seems so flagrant at the present time.

CHAPTER I

NERVOUS FUNCTIONING AND THE BRAIN

WITHOUT dwelling on the origins of the nervous apparatus[1] we may note that at an early stage of its differentiation, when it first constitutes a nervous 'system' capable of ensuring individuality of behaviour in multicellular organisms, three kinds of cell elements appear: receptive,[2] motor, and connective. By the morphological grouping of elements of the same category motor and connecting centres, also called centres of reflex activity, may be formed.

It is the connective elements which truly characterize nervous function; at this level enter the extraneous dynamogenic or inhibitory influences, and here too the influence arises which can carry the activation or the inhibition elsewhere. And it is these reciprocal influences, favourable or preventive, which produce the co-ordination involved in animal individuality.

This co-ordination is susceptible of degrees like the individuality to which it gives rise. The sea-urchin which Uexküll calls "a republic of reflexes" has a co-ordination less definite than the star-fish, in which we find that peculiar form of co-ordination with unequal powers known as subordination, though it is a subordination still variable and momentary. In such an

[1] On the first stages of nervous differentiation, see G. H. Parker's excellent study, *The Elementary Nervous System* (Monographs on Experimental Biology), 1919.

[2] The central receptive element must be distinguished from the sensory peripheral neurone which is a true receptor organ, analogous to the muscle, a reacting organ.

organism, consisting of a star with almost identical arms, any arm can be the directing influence, and no one of them is necessarily or always so; the power of directing the general locomotion of the organism belongs at any given moment to the arm which receives from the outside world the greatest sum of excitations, and thus possesses a higher dynamogeny.

In an annelid worm the morphological arrangement fixes the directive power in a particular region, which possesses sense organs peculiar to itself, as well as motor and grasping organs and the mechanism of mastication and suction situated round the entrance to the digestive tube. This is the cephalic region in which important motor and sensory centres, and correlative connecting centres are collected for the functions of these organs of movement and sensation. Thus the brain has become a predominant organ, but its predominance varies greatly with the species.

Without pausing to inquire into the various degrees of this cerebral pre-eminence, we will proceed at once to the most complex forms of the nervous system, in order to rediscover there the fundamental elements presented by the simplest forms, which correspond to reception, distribution and discharge.

In the organization of a mammal we find on the one hand receptor elements — besides the peripheral neurones of the spinal ganglia—grouped in the posterior horns of the spinal cord and in the bulbar nuclei; on the other hand we have motor elements in the anterior horns and the bulbar nuclei, all forming segmentary centres which fuse in a continuous column penetrating the skull; and there, as part of the encephalon or of the brain in the broad sense, are found the receptor elements of the cutaneous surfaces and the deep regions of the head, and the motor elements of the cephalic muscles.

Between the receptor and motor elements there are connecting elements which form the reflex centres.

If, in the case of man, the skin of the sole of the foot be rubbed with the head of a pin, the toes flex. The stimulus elaborated by the peripheral neurones located in the spinal ganglion is transmitted to receptor elements situated in the posterior horns of the spinal cord at the

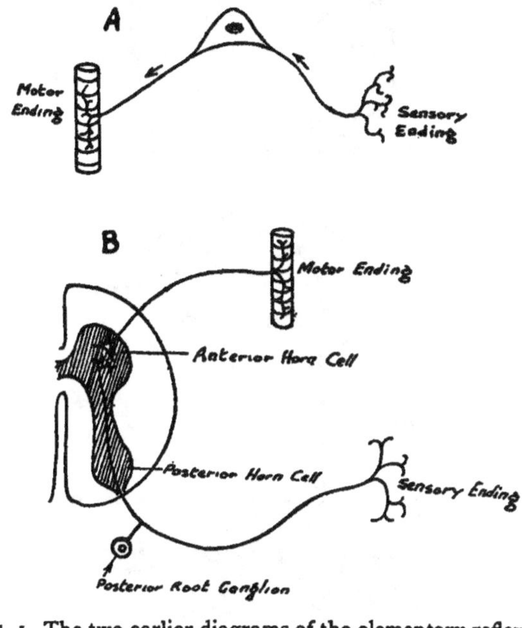

FIG. 1. The two earlier diagrams of the elementary reflex.

A. (Diagram of Küss and Duval in 1872). A single nerve cell connects the sensory and motor end-organs.

B. (Diagram of current physiological text-books). The stimulus received by the sensory cell in the posterior root ganglion penetrates the posterior horn cell of the spinal cord and is connected with the motor cell of the anterior horn cell.

level of the first sacral segment, and then to the connecting element which form a reflex centre and are located in this lumbo-sacral region. Hence a stimulus is transmitted to the motor centres of the flexor muscles of the toes, in the anterior homolateral horns of this same medullary level.

We are here dealing with a simple reflex, but there are

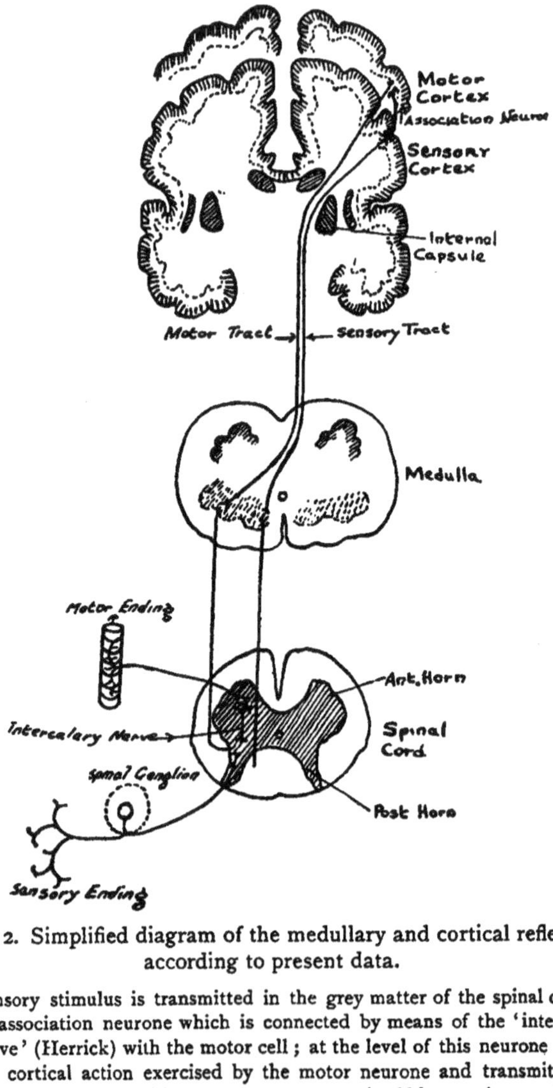

FIG. 2. Simplified diagram of the medullary and cortical reflexes according to present data.

The sensory stimulus is transmitted in the grey matter of the spinal cord to an association neurone which is connected by means of the 'intercalary nerve' (Herrick) with the motor cell; at the level of this neurone begins the cortical action exercised by the motor neurone and transmitted by the motor tract. This motor neurone may itself be put into action by the sensory impulse which follows the sensory tract after crossing the neuronic relays (only the bulbar nucleus of which is indicated) by means of the association neurones.

complex reflexes demanding the co-ordination of movements, such as the reflex of the decerebrate frog, which will use its foot to wipe a drop of acid from a spot on the skin. In the case of man, after an upper medullary section which is physiologically adequate, a moderate stimulation of the sole of the foot will provoke the withdrawal of the lower limb stimulated by the combined action of a whole group of muscles, and the extension of the lower limb on the other side; the outline of a co-ordinated walking-movement is produced, as, in the case of Sherrington's 'spinal' dog—that is to say a dog whose spinal cord alone was functioning—similar movements are produced by a medullary automatism under the influence of very varied excitations. There is in the spinal cord a connecting centre of more complex action which may be called a *co-ordination centre.* This centre governs the inhibition and activation of a great number of muscles, in such a way as to bring about alternate harmonic movements. It receives indications from the receptive centres, governs the individual activity of the various motor centres, and also acts on the elementary connecting centres.

In the upper regions of the cerebro-spinal axis there are analogous centres which govern the combined movements of the head and eyes. And it is the existence of these co-ordinating centres which is of primary importance in nervous functioning, and particularly in cerebral functioning.

But before dealing with the brain, it is well to distinguish a second characteristic of nervous organization which renders it an organization in levels.

A rough comparison may help to explain this organization.

Imagine a commercial house or an agency containing a central office in which some of the employees are engaged in receiving telephone messages, each in communication with a single exterior station, others in transmitting orders, each also in communication with a single executive station; and further, a number of persons appointed to carry out the orders, each in touch with several receivers and several employees who are transmitters only. Here we have an outline of the elementary form of nervous centralization.

The service develops and complications arise; to give orders it is sometimes necessary to consult the records, to take a large number of facts into account, and to delay or accelerate the execution of other orders. In some cases a very urgent response is necessary, a response which is always the same and which requires no preliminary deliberation. The original office is retained, but higher floors are added, containing more receiving employees, transmitting employees, individuals charged with the elaboration of orders, and finally a particularly large number of employees to act as connecting agents. These put the chiefs into communication with one another, and, above all, see to it that each is in possession of any information likely to be of use to him, and make it their particular business to communicate as required the whole of the data collected by the receiving agents. Finally, they consult the records.

Let us assume that there are four or five floors, the most complete organization is on the top, the intermediate floors being more or less analogous to the original office.[1]

When information arrives, it is received by an agent in the office below, who transmits it to a connecting agent of his office, and also to the receiving agent in the office above, who likewise sends it on until it reaches the highest floor.

Certain messages require a simple immediate response, indicated by the connecting agent below to his transmitting employees, but others necessitate a more com-

[1] The last stage is not merely a terminal receptor but a reacting organ; for the whole of the nervous apparatus forms a cyclic system; if there is not occasionally a motor reaction, reflex or elaborated, there will at any rate be a mental and associative reaction with inhibitory consequences functionally equivalent to the motor impulses.

plex elaboration. When they reach the connecting agent, who responds automatically and without reflecting, this agent, in consequence of precautions taken by the transmitting agents on the upper floors, is prevented from communicating with his own transmitting agents. The inhibition may bear upon his apparatus of communication or upon the apparatus of the transmitting agents, or again it may affect the path of communication, and this may be practically broken.

The news is transmitted upwards from floor to floor; if the connecting elements of the intermediate floors are equally inhibited, the order required by this information will receive considerable elaboration in the light of information already received, at the same time or later, by various receptive agents at the first station, and likewise communicated from floor to floor; and this order will then be communicated, directly this time and without delay at the intermediate floors, to the transmitting agents below, who alone are in communication with the outside world.

We know, in fact, that every sensory impulse must traverse a series of neuronic relays before reaching the cerebral cortex, and there are also cortical cells, described as motor, which are particularly voluminous (Betz' cells); these send their axis-cylinder by the pyramidal tract to the direct motor neurones of the anterior horns of the spinal cord, without passing through an intermediate station.

The reflex responses which originate at different levels cannot all be equally inhibited by the action of the higher centres. Take the case of a hot or even burning object touching the hand; if, for reasons furnished by other sensory impressions or by the associative evocation of memories or ideas, the organism of the final stage decides that none the less the hand shall remain motionless, it will inhibit the regular withdrawal reflex of a 'spinal' animal; but whether voluntary or not, there will always be marked local vaso-dilatation. If the stimulus is sufficiently painful owing to the influence of the reflex centre at the thalamic level, there will be a pupillary dilatation, a modification of blood pressure, and a whole series of visceral reactions. These reactions would, however, generally be more intense if the reflex centre were completely separated from the top floor of the edifice, which exerts a constant moderating influence, even on the system known as the 'vegetative life,' and is in closer relation than we sometimes think with integrative action.[1]

We thus get an idea of the way in which the nervous system functions in the highest organisms, the cerebral hemispheres representing the higher floor, the intermediate brain and the middle brain corresponding to the other floors, and finally the lower station continuing along the length of the bulb and the spinal cord.

But in this rough outline a special place must be assigned to the agents which correspond to the *co-ordinating* elements and centres.

When complex actions occur, and when these responses are produced frequently enough, the order is not directly communicated to the various interested transmitting agents, but passes, with suitable instructions, by means of an employee specialized for the transmission of this particular order, and possessing an apparatus which he has already prepared and which allows him by pressing once upon a key to achieve the complete transmission automatically. Thus, an order to look to the right will involve the intervention of co-ordinating agents in close connection with each other, and these will call into play the transmitting

[1] The general inhibitory and regulative action of the higher centres increases with the differentiation of the system: and hence, in the dog and especially in man, we find a strong inhibition of gastric movements, psychical in origin. This inhibition is very weak in the guinea-pig, though it is even revealed by decerebration; in the case of the tortoise, too, decerebration is followed by a slight acceleration of the movements of the stomach, but not so with the frog, where this inhibitory influence is lacking altogether.

agents of certain muscles of the neck and of the eyes, in such a way that the head will turn towards the right and both eyes will turn in the same direction. This implies that the right internal muscle of the right eye must relax and the right external muscle contract, while the right external muscle of the left eye will relax and the right internal muscle contract with an intensity regulated by the stimulation of the retina caused by the movement itself. This inverse play between the two pairs of antagonistic muscles of the two sides of the body is produced rapidly and accurately, thanks to the co-ordinating (oculodextrogyric) agent for right ocular movements, while a movement to the left will be ensured by another agent (oculolaevogyric) for left ocular movements. The independence of these two agents has been clearly shown by pathological research.[1]

A reflex order from the penultimate floor, a voluntary order elaborated by the higher administrative bureaux and creating a tendency to look to the right or the left, will only be executed by means of the indispensable co-ordinating agent.

The agents of ocular movement are predetermined by the hereditary organization, in the structural plan, as it were, of man's nervous system. But, when frequently repeated movements become habitual, new co-ordinating agents are established; so that a skilful cyclist, when he feels in danger of falling to one side,

[1] By an ingenious comparison, de Lapersonne and Cantonnet explain the arrangement of this apparatus as follows: "Consider the two eye-balls as two horses attached to the same carriage; the pole which separates them represents the median plane of the body; each horse is guided by a right rein and a left rein (each rein represents a muscle, a nerve and its primary nucleus). The right rein of each horse unites with the right rein of the other horse to constitute the common right rein held by the right hand of the coachman; the same is true for the two left reins uniting in a common left rein held by the left hand of the coachman. The right hand of the coachman is the co-ordinating centre for right ocular movements (for it controls the peripheral apparatus, the right reins, which direct the two horses to the right): his left hand is the co-ordinating centre for left ocular movements" (*Manuel de neurologie oculaire*, pp. 42-43).

rights himself through the intervention of co-ordinating agents which, as soon as they are warned, will at once bring about the movements of the arms necessary to balance the machine. Moreover, when the movements necessary for a given receptive reaction are constantly repeated in the same form, the reaction becomes a reflex and can be effected at an intermediate stage without reference to the superior service. There is a shortening of the paths, and certain reactions will still be possible even when an accident has prevented the reception at the last stage. This is an important point, and it enables us to explain certain rather perplexing facts of cerebral physiology, as we shall see somewhat later.

Let us now, while keeping closely in touch with physiological data, try to determine the main lines of the functioning of the upper level, in so far as we can know anything of it, whether by introspection or more especially by such objective information as can be obtained, thanks to language, from the examination both of normal men and of those affected by various cerebral disturbances.

Chapter II

MENTAL FUNCTIONING AND THE BRAIN

The excitation of a peripheral sensory apparatus, a tactile corpuscle for example, provokes a particular sensation, and no other stimulus, even that of an analogous corpuscle differently situated, will give the same sensation. Similarly, the appearance of a light whose image is thrown on a particular point of the retina will give a particular sensation, while an analogous excitation of any other part of the body will either give no sensation at all or one that is analogous but not identical—as in the case of the excitation of another retinal area.

Each peripheral sensory apparatus gives rise to special sensations; it can produce not one kind of sensation only—differing in intensity alone—but several; in one point of the retina, for example, excitations may arise capable of producing various sensations of colour. Each peripheral apparatus, tactile corpuscle, retinal rod or cone, olfactory glomerulus, etc. is in connection with one or several cortical cells like so many bells that can respond by a single sound, which is the specific sensation. If we can bring these terminal cells into play by any process other than the normal physiological process, by electrical stimulation of the nerve fibres which connect them with the peripheral apparatus, or by direct excitation—electrical stimulation of the cortex, mechanical shock, chemical irritation, etc.—we shall cause the bells to ring and shall evoke the specific sensations of the cortical elements stimulated. Many facts may be adduced in support of this specificity of cortical responses, to which J. Müller's doctrine of the specific energy of the nerves may be reduced.

The sensation aroused is accompanied more or less definitely by an affective impression, agreeable or disagreeable, which may assume the more complex appearance of an emotion such as fear or anger, linked to multiple reactions and in particular to a form of motor behaviour, oscillating between the two poles of flight and aggression.

This affective repercussion seems to take place at the penultimate stage of the nervous system and governs complicated reflexes or instinctive reactions.

Normally, however, affective impressions are controlled by groups of sensations which constitute perceptions: chromatic sensations, of a red tonality, arranged in a certain manner and distributed so that they correspond to rounded forms, provoke the perception of a cherry. To perceive a cherry is to recognize it; the perception involves mnemonic data. It is because the sensory group has already occurred several times and has been followed by various events, themselves the object of sensations, that the reappearance of this group, which tends to re-awaken the memory of the same events, the reproduction of the same acts, is recognized. Conversely, the image of the cherry could itself be evoked by the perception or the memory of subsequent events (for example the fact of eating the cherry and spitting out the stone).

The image of the cherry acquires at the same time, by the repetition of experiences, an ever greater evocative power and an ever easier evocability. This fact of perception provides the key to the phenomena of memory.

Memory, in fact, is nothing but the reinforcement and facilitation of the passage of the nervous impulse along certain paths.

To recall a sensation is to make use of a beaten path

conducting a cerebral nervous impulse to a cortical sensory bell, which is made to sound without waiting for the intervention of an external stimulus; the elementary sensory image does not differ from the sensation, save in the manner in which it is provoked, and generally in intensity, which is much less except when toxic irritation or inflammation augments the response of the specific bell and renders it pathologically hyper-excitable.

The complex image of the object will not differ essentially from the perceptive grouping: the elementary sensations—or at least some of them—will be called up simultaneously or successively under the conditions and in the order in which this natural evocation by adequate external stimuli has become habitual; and from the evocation and revival of this group will arise impulses evocative of other groups and other images by mnemonic action, according to the paths involved.

Memory does not reside in the image considered as a static whole, but in the dynamic power of reconstituting the perception, whose elements are nothing but sensations, revived and aroused by a stimulus of central origin in place of the habitual peripheral excitation, and equally capable of being provoked by an artificial electrical stimulus, if we could limit this stimulus to the required cortical cells.

The play of sensations, since it involves the repetition of numerous experiences, involves also the formation of familiar association paths by the application of a general law of neurophysiology, of which memory represents only one particular case.

When one perception has just been produced—that of a cherry for example—these association paths lead to evocations of sensations or rather groups of sensations, that is to say of images, and lead also to reactions which are conditioned not only by mnemonic facilitation, as in the case of reflexes, but by variable influences. These influences arrive from various groups of sensations perceived simultaneously, and in particular internal sensations constituting coenesthesia; they also arrive from affective impressions endowed with a motor power so that they are often confused with tendencies, that is to say with the outline of the reaction which they control, and these affective impressions play an important part from the point of view of the liberation of reactive nervous energy.

The sight of the cherry, when the organism is in a given condition, will provoke an intense emotion, which appears as an impulse, a desire; and with the aid of abundant associative stimuli it will produce actions calculated to satisfy this desire. The desired actions will be realized by means of impulses coming from cortical incitor elements. The functioning of these nervous elements, which give rise to movements by means of motor elements proper, or of subordinate co-ordinating centres at a lower level, to which suitable orders will be supplied, will reappear subjectively as a peculiar impression, an impression of volition linked with their activity.

If, as in an experiment which has been recorded,[1] we provoke the functioning of these cortical elements by electrical stimulation—replacing the nervous impulse of central origin—in a conscious subject whose brain is exposed, he will imagine that he is himself directing the movement, though, in fact, it is beyond his control.

In general a volitional act does not imply the simple contraction of an isolated muscle, and the incitation of an elementary group of medullary motor cells: there is a group of simultaneous and successive contractions,

[1] *Cf.* Harvey Cushing, "A Note upon the Faradic Stimulation of the Postcentral Gyrus in Conscious Patients," *Brain*, XXXII., 1, 1909, p. 44. Observations made on a boy of 15 who was aware of the movements provoked by direct electrical stimulation of the cortex, and had a feeling that these movements were produced by him in response to peripheral stimulation; he had a sensation of active muscular contraction, altogether different from that accompanying a contraction caused by electrical stimulation of the motor nerve.

whose arrangement and order are determined by the bringing into play of the appropriate incitor elements.

Here too memory intervenes—in the form generally known as habit—gradually facilitating by repetition the functional evocation of volitions in the arrangement and order which correspond to the realization of the complex act.

The question may be raised whether each of the cortical incitor elements, the volitional elements, is in connection, by means of the motor medullary agent, with a given muscle; or whether they are co-ordinating elements whose incitation is complex, each ensuring the contraction of certain muscles and the relaxation of certain others by a single action, in such a way as to secure the realization of some movement, such as the closing of the fist, or at any rate the flexing of the fingers. Since we find that even the movements of walking are controlled by the medullary co-ordination centres, it may be assumed that movements — or at any rate simple movements—are 'willed' by single cortical elements. In fact we cannot dissociate at will the play of certain muscles. The centres of the cortex which we call 'motor' are in reality elementary co-ordinating centres.

But in actions which are somewhat complex, the incitor elements themselves must behave according to a certain arrangement and in a certain order.

In the case of really complicated actions, very frequently repeated, may not some part be played by special co-ordinating centres themselves capable of inciting the inciting centres, according to a fixed schema exemplified by the lower stages? There is no doubt that this does, in fact, occur. For speech, writing, musical execution, for every complex operation of a motor apparatus intended to produce precise actions that could be the object of a single volition such as the pronouncing or writing of a word, the playing of a note or a group of notes, etc. we have to suppose that there are central relay stations where, for a given volition, a corresponding intermediary will be responsible for bringing the cortical incitor elements into play at a single stroke, by means of a sort of switch-board prepared in advance and corresponding to the motor set. These are the dynamic sets which are realized by the co-ordinating centres and are generally called motor images—an ambiguous term that lends itself to endless confusion. We shall have to return to these points.

The co-ordination centre is a station which, at the entrance of the incito-motor area of the cortex, receives certain familiar associative orders that are difficult to execute, and ensures their rapid and exact performance. It is probable that similar intermediary agents are also to be found for the centres we call sensory, whose function is to arouse associative reactions rather than automatic reflexes, and which may be called 'incito-associative.'

We may note that certain perceptions and certain images acquire, by repetition and use, an exceptional practical value and evocative power. These are 'symbols,' and they may be substituted for a great number of particular images which they can replace through their associative power, for the provocation of other images or oppropriate reactions.

Consider hieroglyphic symbols and printed signs in black on white, such as are perceived in reading this page. These signs, though very similar, may yet have very different evocative power; and if this power irradiated directly from the cortical receptive elements it would entail an immense complication and entanglement of tracts.

In reality, this grouping of sensations which corresponds to a written image, to the image of a word, will in the case of an educated man who has read and thought much, come into contact, in an intermediate centre, with a single relay element, by which the evocative irradiations will be produced.

Such a centre acts as a co-ordination centre, which, for those schemata to which it is adapted, responds immediately by definite associations; that is to say, opens the association paths peculiar to each schema, and certain of these tracts lead to incito-motor centres.

For example, if I hear the word cherry, this complex auditory impression is transmitted to a co-ordination centre of the auditory schemata; here, a syntonized agent representing the cherry schema will establish, among other multiple connections, the junction with an agent, or schema, of the verbal co-ordinating centre or word-activating centre; and this again will bring into play a vocal group reproducing in speech the word which has been heard.

Thus, on the one hand, sensory impressions terminate in cortical centres, where they produce varied associative incitations by means—in the case of those which come from common objects—of co-ordination centres which come into play as soon as the sensory group corresponding to such an object has been perceived; and on the other hand, among the associations evoked there are some which end, with comparative directness, in provoking movements by the involvement of the incito-motor centres. In every-day actions, this is accomplished by means ef co-ordinating centres which ensure the execution of the required act as soon as they are activated by an associative impulse terminating there.

Between these two stages occur all the intricacies of 'thought.'

In what does this consist?

There can be no question here of magnifying and examining the difficult and complex problem of Thought under the microscope of the interest that we bring to it, for we should soon be irretrievably lost in the maze; in order to connect this function with its organ we must look at it from a sufficient distance to be aware only of its main lines. Moreover, it is necessary to distinguish elementary forms of thought, as we recognize them in the higher animals, from complex forms or symbolic thought, elaborated by a long process of social evolution.

In its elementary form, thought represents nothing more than the successive evocation, by the action of mnemonic machinery, of sensory impressions revived with relative incompleteness—images such as we have defined. The orientation of the evocative associations is constantly governed by a group of factors which include: past experience, with its reinforcement of habitual tracts; present experience, with its totality or sensory data from which a resultant drive emerges; above all, the affective state, with its system of alert tendencies; and finally, the organic state itself, with its circulatory, metabolic or other characteristics, capable of favouring or opposing progress along certain cerebral tracts.

Into the influence of past experience enters the mechanism of symbolic thought, the contribution of social education; language is the principal form of symbolization, and it allows us to sum up and condense the results obtained by the thought of successive generations, and even to direct, according to imperative rules—especially the rules of logic and morality—the play of individual association.

The appearance of symbolism renders the sensory basis of thought much less apparent, for the attention is concerned with the evocative power of the symbol much more than by the sensory form in which it is evoked, which is of secondary importance, whether it be purely visual, auditory, or kinesthetic, or mixed. But can the sensory basis be completely lacking? The problem has given rise to much controversy, and the discussion of 'imageless thought' is not yet closed. We will return to this interesting question, but first we must indicate the significance of the idea of a co-ordination centre in the physiological interpretation of the mechanism of language.

The very use of language implies the development of

co-ordination centres which, though doubtless partly prepared by hereditary transmission in our old-established civilizations, are developed by individual education: auditory co-ordination centres and, when education is complete, visual (or tactile among the blind) on the sensory side; vocal, or (in deaf mutes) mimicry, co-ordination centres, and, when education is complete, graphic centres, on the incito-motor side.

The rôle of the co-ordination centres becomes predominant with the play of symbols whose mutual evocation constitutes abstract thought; in abstract thought the evocation does not necessarily lead to the images which give a meaning to the symbols. Each symbol has an evocative capacity for images which is more extensive, but also less exact, according as the symbol, the concept, is more abstract and general; the outline of the evocation, of whose facility we are informed by special feelings, will be sufficient. Furthermore, there are even symbols of symbols, evocative of images only in the second degree, by means of primary stations of the co-ordination centres.

Great individual differences naturally appear in these forms of complex thoughts, both as regards the evocation of images and the mere interplay of symbolic associations. In the latter case, they vary according to the predominance of the auditory, visual, or sometimes tactile, symbols, or even of motor schemata often accompanied by the beginnings of motor realization, which produce corresponding sensations.

One person will think especially with the co-ordination centres of visual imagery, elementary co-ordination centres for the vision of objects, verbal co-ordination centres in the case of reading, and will make more frequent appeal to concrete images which he will call up and place, and which will help him in his intellectual activity; another will 'think aloud' in so far as motor assistance is necessary to him; yet another will hear his internal thought as a conversation, using only auditory verbal images which arise at the call of the co-ordination centres.

The thought of the painter, the musician, the geometrician, the tradesman, and the philosopher may take very different forms; still more so the thought of the uncultivated man, which remains rudimentary and revolves for ever in the same circles.

Thought is dynamic and associative. And it is clear, too, that the exercise of thought requires numerous association paths, which are more numerous according as it is more fertile, linking up, with various relay elements and shunts, the receptive stations, the incito-motor stations, and their co-ordination centres, and, in particular, linking the numerous agents of these stations in an infinite number of ways.

And we see, in fact, that the progress of intelligence among the vertebrates runs parallel with the development of the association paths. Even if we rule out everything to do with the receptive and incito-motor stations, which require a greater number of agents in proportion as the body, with its surfaces of reception or of reaction, increases in size, we find that there remains in the various animal species a part of the brain—which is properly associative—independent of the animal's size and very characteristic of the intellectual level of the species.

And even among the invertebrates we can discover in the higher species, especially the Cephalopoda and social Hymenoptera, important nervous areas which serve neither for reception nor motor incitation, that is to say projection, nor even as simple synapses; and these, being situated at a higher level and replete with complex association paths, should make possible some form of thought, such as is indicated by the marked capacity of the species in question (devil-fish, bee, or ant, for example) to profit by experience and to adapt its behaviour to circumstances.

CHAPTER III

THE PROBLEM OF LOCALIZATION

CAN we regard the nervous apparatus of the cerebral cortex, which constitutes the highest stage of the directive system of the organism, as undifferentiated to such a degree that a lesion, wherever it occurred, would only diminish its functional capacity as a whole; and, in proportion to the extent of the injury, would involve a constant succession of disturbances disappearing in a precisely inverse order with the progress of recovery? Or should we rather expect to find in the various regions of the cortex individualized centres grouped in departments with well-defined functions, and endeavour to localize memory, intelligence, attention, morality, æsthetics, loyalty, musical talent, or aptitude for mathematics?

Neither of these extreme positions is in agreement with the facts of cerebral anatomico-physiology or with the conditions of nervous and mental functioning. Let us start from a study of these conditions, and note roughly what we can learn from the facts, and particularly what we owe to war pathology; and, first of all, let us examine what we know of local differentiation of the incito-associative receptive function, of the incito-motor reactive function, and of the co-ordinative functions, before penetrating into the mazes of the associative functions and the complexities of thought.

1. *Incito-Associative Receptor Centres*

Experiments on the higher vertebrates, on highly evolved mammals, dogs, cats and monkeys, have given evidence of regions in the cerebral cortex which are affected by the reception of various kinds of sensations; an ablation of the occipital area renders the animals blind, a double temporal ablation renders them deaf. Their behaviour is no longer modified by visual experience in one case or of auditory experience in the other.

These localizations did, it is true, receive a rude shock when it was noticed that an animal trained to react in a certain way to a given noise could still do so correctly after the extirpation of the auditory cortical areas, and that it can still even be trained to take its food at an auditory signal. But Kalischer's[1] experiments on the dog were repeated after a more complete destruction of the cortical areas, and under more rigid experimental conditions, with precisely opposite results.[2]

In mammals with a more rudimentary nervous system, such as rats, it certainly seems that habits acquired on a sensory basis could be effectively realized in the absence of the greater part of the cerebral cortex, and in particular, after the ablation of the areas regarded as receptive.[3]

The development of centralization, which is correlated with cerebral evolution, does not allow the inference from a particular functional distribution in a given animal species to the same distribution in a different species.

The part played by the first relay centres, along the receptive tracts, is the more important according as the terminal station is less developed. This terminal station, in mammals, extends into the covering of the telencepha-

[1] "Zur Funktion des Schläfenlappens des Grosshirns," *Sitzungsber, der K. Ak. der Wiss. Berlin*, 1907, p. 204. *Cf.* also *Arch. für Phys.*, 1909, p. 303.

[2] *Cf.* Rothmann, "Uber die Ergebnisse der Hörprüfung an dressierten Hunden," *Arch. für Physiol.*, 1908, p. 107.

[3] *Cf.* K. S. Lashley, "Studies of Cerebral Function in Learning," *Psychobiology*, 1920, II, pp. 55-135 (Researches of S. I. Franz and Lashley. *Cf. Psychobiology*, 1917, I, pp. 3-18 and 71-134).

lon, the cerebral cortex of the hemispheres folded and convoluted to occupy the greatest possible surface in the cranial box; and in the birds it reaches as far as the telencephalic floor in the striate body.[1] It must not be forgotten that most fishes have, properly speaking, no cerebral cortex, and that their more simple behaviour is governed altogether by the first receptive stations, although no fundamental difference separates them from the vertebrates which possess a cortex.

The functioning of the relay centres is inhibited to a great extent by the action of the terminal station, which is in constant relation with them; but they always retain a certain autonomy, even in the higher mammals, and in man.

Thus the closing of the eyelids under the sudden influence of a bright light can still occur in the case of a cat or a dog deprived of its entire cerebral cortex, or only of the occipital area that serves for visual reception;[2] but the general behaviour of the organism is not influenced by the light. There is real blindness (Dusser de Barenne).

In man, this dissociation of the reflex function and of the associative function in connection with sensory reception is evident, if not in the case of the dazzle reflex controlled by the terminal station, at least in the case of pupillary contraction occasioned by light. When an occipital lesion has caused total blindness but the sub-cortical centres have not themselves been injured either directly or indirectly, we find that the pupillary reflex

[1] *Cf.* G. Kalischer, *Das Grosshirn der Papageien in anatomischer und physiologischer Beziehung*, 1905 (Anhang zu den Abh. der kön. Ak. der Wissensch.).

[2] When only the 'visual' cerebral area is absent, the dazzle reflex may be lacking (Minkowski), though not when the decerebration is more complete, provided the sub-cortical centres are untouched. This is because a lesion, we shall later have occasion to observe, involves disturbing functioual imbalances, and the imbalance is more marked in a partial injury to the superior centre than in its suppression as a whole (*cf.* Dusser de Barenne, "Recherches expérimentales sur les fonctions du systeme nerveux central," *Arch. néerl. de Physiol.*, 1919, p. 13).

persists, which is a sign of the integrity—or at any rate the relative integrity—of the retina and the optic tracts.

Such pathological data are of vital importance for the study of the human brain. Owing to the considerable differences in the degree of functional centralization found in the other species, experimental physiology is unable to settle the problem of functional localization in the cortex, even for sensory receptions. Pathology, with its unprepared experiments, must provide almost all the necessary data, though anatomy offers some assistance, in tracing the course of the connecting tracts.

Pathology has confirmed the experiments on mammals, and shows that the reception of cutaneous and kinesthetic sensibility for the entire body takes place in the ascending parietal convolution just behind the fissure of Rolando, that the reception of auditory sensations takes place in the temporal lobe, and finally that the reception of visual sensations is accomplished in the occipital lobe.[1]

Lesions of the brain due to bullets and bursting shells during the War have confirmed these data and increased their accuracy; but they do not seem to have furnished clear information in the matter of gustatory and olfactory sensations, to which little attention has been devoted, and whose probable seat lies in regions less exposed to limited lesions compatible with survival; nor have they provided any useful information as regards auditory localization. In fact, each peripheral auditory system appears to be connected with both cerebral hemispheres, so that a lesion limited to one hemisphere of the receptive area does not involve deafness, since the other hemisphere continues to ensure the auditory sensitivity of both ears. A destruction of both temporal auditory areas is necessary in order to

[1] The cortical centre of vision was discovered by Panizza in 1856, and is one of the many notable achievements of Italian physiology, to which we owe so much of our knowledge of nervous functions.

bring about immediate deafness: in fact cortical deafness of one ear only is unknown.

When we turn to vision matters are somewhat different. The two right hemi-retinæ which ensure the vision of the left part of the field are in connection with the right hemisphere, and the two left hemi-retinæ with the left hemisphere. The destruction of a receptive centre, right or left, involves hemianopsia, blindness limited to the left or right field of vision.[1]

But the war lesions added greatly to our knowledge of the exact topography of the visual centres, which were very often injured, sometimes in a very small area, by a tiny shell-splinter, for example.

It has been definitely established that the two hemiretinæ are superimposed by parallel projection on the surface of the occipital visual area which surrounds the calcarine fissure, so that a partial destruction in this region of the cortex involves a corresponding binocular scotoma in the visual field for all forms of sensibility to light and colour. The situation and size of this gap is determined by the seat and extent of the injury.

We shall return later to these facts, which provide an excellent example of the precision with which the projections of the sensory peripheral surfaces can be localized in the receptive station of the cortex.

As regards the centres of cutaneous and deep sensibility which are the chief object of controversy, the war cases also provide important data. The principal results can be stated, and they agree with certain recent tendencies and with numerous facts already established, as we shall see in greater detail in Part II.

The cutaneous surface, like the retinal surface, is projected on the cerebral cortex, this time along the ascending parietal convolution behind the fissure of Rolando. Each half of the body is found on the opposite hemisphere, the lower limb above and the

[1] Hemianopsia was discovered by Munk and also, independently, in 1879, by Luciani and Tamburini.

cephalic region below. The cortical area occupied by a cutaneous surface varies in size with the sensibility of this surface, that is to say there is a greater density of peripheral arrangements, of innervation fibres; thus the hand occupies a considerable area, and is therefore more easily affected. There are also topographical groupings, two of which are for the limbs and are quite distinct though contiguous, roughly representing two

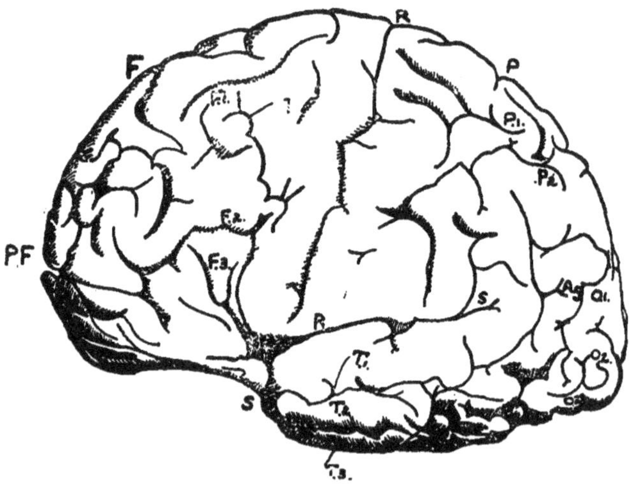

FIG. 3. Lateral surface of the left hemisphere (Debierre).

S. Sylvian fissure. R. Fissure of Rolando. F. Frontal lobe (convolutions F^1, F^2 and F^3). A.f. Ascending frontal (or pre-Rolandic or first central or antero-central convolution). A.p. Ascending parietal (or post-Rolandic or second central or central posterior convolution). P. Parietal lobe (convolutions P^1 and P^2). O. Occipital lobe (convolutions O^1, O^2 and O^3). T. Temporal lobe (convolutions T^1, T^2 and T^3). A.g. Angular gyrus.

longitudinal halves. In particular the representation of a half-hand, the thumb and index side, is found to be distinct from that of the other half, the ulnar side, the localization for each being at a different level, along the fissure.

Deep sensibility, particularly kinesthetic sensibility, is in juxtaposition with the forms of cutaneous sensibility for each region of the body, the sensibility of the half-hands to movements being in the same area as the various cutaneous sensibilities (temperature and touch); they are not situated, as has been claimed, in the motor area.

Certain facts have, however, suggested that the deeper sensations may be located elsewhere, in the parietal region: and lesions of the parietal lobe do, in fact, often involve disturbances of deep sensibility. But

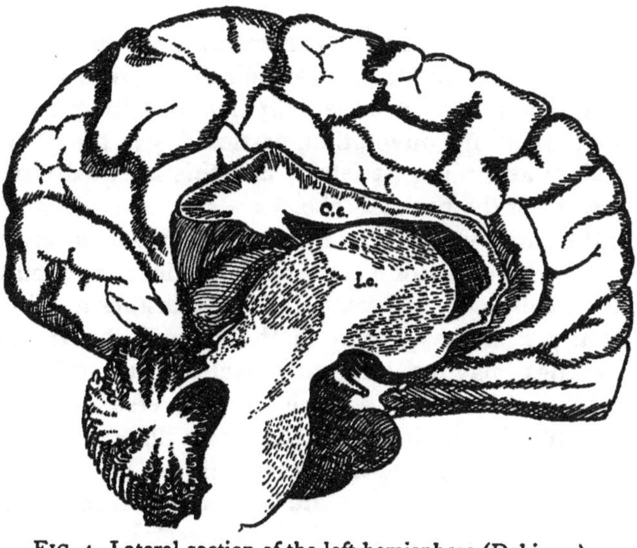

FIG. 4. Lateral section of the left hemisphere (Debierre).
C.c. Corpus callosum (interhemispheric commissure). I.c. Internal capsule.

this is an error of the same order as the location of these sensibilities further in front of the cutaneous area, in the ascending frontal, which is a motor region.

To understand how this error arose we must recall the nature of the disturbances which can result from cerebral lesions. These are of three types: they may consist in an irritation (the beginning of an inflammatory process, for example) and involve hallucinatory processes in the sensory centres and exaggerated reactions to slight irritations, usually accompanied by disturbances of perception; or they may involve destruction with complete functional suppression, limited to the area destroyed, involving for example total and definitive hemianopsic blindness; or finally, they may represent a functional inhibition, a constraint producing suppression, which is generally incomplete but of diffuse boundaries and rather widespread. This disturbance, which is often found in cases of shock, usually complicates the localized destruction and seems to increase its territory.

A destructive lesion of the motor area in the first central convolution or the ascending frontal is accompanied by a disturbance that may suppress functions in the neighbouring convolution, particularly in the second central (or ascending parietal); and this is equally true for lesions of the parietal lobe.

In the same way a very limited destructive lesion of the receptive area of cutaneous and deep sensibility often involves a generalized hemianæsthesia which gradually decreases. But in these cases the various sensibilities may be unequally excited, and this dissociation, which may assume very diverse forms, is responsible for the idea that there is a different topography for the centres of these sensibilities.

In reality the disorders are rendered diffuse by the reverberation of comparatively distant destructive lesions which may be insignificant; total functional suppression then rarely occurs and the rate at which it more or less completely disappears varies with the distance between the area affected and the area directly injured. There are varied hypoæsthesias, but certain forms of sensibility are generally more susceptible. Thus colour vision, or chromatic sensibility, is always suppressed more quickly than light vision, and is the last to return.

The mechanism of this distant reverberation from a central lesion cannot be accurately determined, and is certainly very complex; mechanical, inflammatory, chemical and vascular phenomena may be involved in varying degrees according to the nature of the lesion (tumour, cyst, hæmorrhage, softening due to the obliteration of nutritive vessels, inflammation of bacterial origin, laceration, etc.). But, in addition, the functional suppression or the acute irritation of a group of neurones may have considerable effect on relatively distant neurones which are in habitual connection with them. A functional imbalance may occur, and its reverberations may be very widespread.

Von Monakow attributed special importance to this idea and bestowed on it a somewhat unfortunate name, which is repellant rather than evocative: he called this functional imbalance of the whole, by a partial disturbance, a "diaschisis." By this he means a well marked syndrome closely related to shock, and representing a sort of local struggle for the maintenance of a disturbed function, with transmission of the disturbance to an element of this complex; it would be characterized especially by temporary paralysis due to the absence of an habitual stimulus (negative inhibition).

If its ordinary relations with one of these connected stations—especially a higher station, upon whose orders it is accustomed to depend—no longer persists, a relay centre, for example, will remain disturbed for a long time, and will no longer fulfil even the functions for which it is autonomous.[1]

The general phenomenon of reverberation at a distance is one of the most important causes of error in attempts at functional nervous localization, and explains many contradictions. The return of vision after complete blindness through occipital lesion or of motor power after total hemiplegia, interpreted as a proof either of substitution or of functional recovery, in spite of the destruction of the corresponding centres, really indicates a temporary disturbance without genuine destruction.

[1] Von Monakow, *Die Lokalisation im Grosshirn*, 1914.—R. Mourgue, "La notion de diaschise et le problème de l'évolution de la fonction dans l'œuvre de Monakow," *L'Encéphale*, 1921, 3.—P. Ladame, "Les Localisations cerébrales d'après Von Monakow," *Revue Neurologique*, 1919, XXVI, pp. 32-40.

Another difficulty lies in the exact determination of the seat and the extent of the lesion: landmarks are necessary and the morphological variability of the brain, in man at any rate, is considerable. On the other hand, the morphological aspect with which we have long been content has no true significance. For it must not be supposed that the distribution of the centres is occasioned by the situation of the convolutions and sulci that characterize the cortical folding of the cerebral hemispheres contained in the cranial box. In fact cerebral architectonics, the histological study of the structure of the layers of the cortex,[1] has established the fact that the functional areas corrrespond to the presence of certain arrangements of cells; and these functional areas have proved capable of considerable individual variation.

Elliot Smith's *area striata*, which constitutes the visual receptive area, has not always precisely the same limits in relation to the convolutions, the more so as the fold itself also varies somewhat in spite of the persistence of the same general design.

The receptive area of the ascending parietal includes the pyramidal cells in deep and intermediate layers in which the sensory tracts end, and which represent particular bells set in motion by the peripheral excitations, resulting in associative reactions in the form of specific sensations. This area sometimes encroaches upon the ascending frontal in front of the fissure of Rolando, and encroaches constantly on the area of the parietal lobe.

It is therefore difficult to fix the exact limits of these centres from pathological data; particularly in war pathology, where a direct examination of the damaged areas after an autopsy was scarcely ever possible. The

[1] "La carte de l'écorce cérébrale," by J. Nageotte (*Revue du mois* VIII, no. 87, 1913, pp. 273-301), lucid and accurate in general arrangement and the work of an histologist who is a biologist in the broad sense, may be profitably consulted.

destructive path was reconstructed and the seat of the lesion indicated by reference to the external point at which the projectile entered, and especially by radiological determination in two planes of the location of the bullet or piece of shell in the brain; and the method adopted gave excellent results.

Though by this means we can obtain coincidences, whose value lies in their repetition, between definite disturbances and the seats of given lesions, it is quite certain that negative cases, in the absence of a microscopic examination to determine the exact seat and extent of the lesion, can have no significance, though they are invariably regarded as important, and sometimes as more important than positive observations.

2. *Incito-motor Centres*

Our knowledge of the region in which the orders that govern the voluntary motor reactions originate was already well advanced when it was supplemented by the contributions of war pathology. The existing data were fully confirmed and no new facts emerged to contradict the established localizations. The incito-motor centres characterized by the presence of giant pyramidal cells (Betz cells), volitional elements in connection with the motor agents of the spinal cord, are arranged in layers along the first central or ascending frontal, in front of the fissure of Rolando, so that from one side of the fissure to the other the receptive area and the motor area are in exact correspondence. Thus a destructive lesion, which bridges the fissure, involves complete anæsthesia and functional paralysis for the same part of the limbs on the other side of the body (for example, the hand and even half the hand); allowing for any disturbances, less complete and more diffuse, due to functional reverberation from the destructive lesion.

But we must also take into account the fact that

cortical paralysis—more or less complete hemiplegia—involves only the suppression of volition, while the actual movements remain possible.[1] Thus a paralysed hand, which cannot be closed voluntarily, closes when the other hand is grasped, through a synergic movement arising from the interaction of the medullary motor centres. So too, hemiplegia of the face prevents voluntary individualized movement, without preventing mimic expression ; and though the closing of the eyelid of the paralysed side only may be impossible, the simultaneous closing of both eyelids, by means of a co-ordination centre at an infra-cortical stage, is perfectly possible.

'Paralysis' of cortical origin is not true paralysis in the sense of a fundamental suppression of motor power, such as may be caused by destruction of the medullary neurones or by section of the motor nerves; it is the paralysis of a certain reactive motor power of the association area;[2] the influence of mental elaboration on motor behaviour in a given organic region ceases after the destruction of the station where the elaborated orders are transmitted.

As the automatic centres, relay co-ordination centres governing certain reaction groups, and the motor centres proper are none of them affected, reflexes and motor associations can always be correctly produced, and even produced with more intensity when they are free from superior inhibitory regulation.

But with the reservation that the volitional centres in the cortex are concerned with certain kinds of movements and are not true motor centres,[3] the stations that we have called incito-motor or associativo-motor are

[1] But the superior lesion may cause functional disorders in the motor centres. This is Von Monakow's "cortico-spinal diaschisis."

[2] We shall see further on that the cortical centres are only incito-motor for certain kinds of movement.

[3] At first, physiologists and pathologists, such as Luciani, thought that the cortical centres were directly motor, to the same degree as the anterior horns of the grey matter, while Pitres and François Franck in France demonstrated their incitatory nature. The rôle of the cortex in epilepsy was at that time under discussion.

now well localized, and the examination of a central lesion in the Rolandic region enables us to foresee the distribution of the paralytic disorders which must result from it.

3. *Receptive Co-ordination Centres*

In considering functional injuries of the receptive centres, we have only examined sensory disturbances, and especially deficiencies (hypo-æsthesia and anæsthesia). Damage to these centres often results, however, in a lack of perception: objects and forms of objects are no longer recognized, for example, when they are felt by the hand; there is an 'astereognosis.'

The stereognostic sense requires the intervention of cutaneous and kinæsthetic sensations, and may disappear when certain component sensations are lacking; but it can disappear independently. Indeed the perceptive function seems, in war lesions, to be more vulnerable and more exposed than the receptive function.

Perception requires the play of associative connections which seem to occur at the level of the most superficial cellular layers of the cortex; and these layers are particularly exposed in lesions of the skull and brain and are often disturbed as a consequence of adjacent destructive lesions. Lesions of the parietal lobe, for example, are generally accompanied by disturbances of tactile perception and astereognosis. Moreover, the mechanism of perceptive association is naturally more delicate than that of reception.

But in addition to diminution of perceptive capacity, there may be total incapacity to recognize objects intellectually; their form may be recognized, but their nature, name and use are not recalled. There is 'agnosia,' which is all the more striking in that it is concerned especially with the most familiar objects, and those most easy to recognize.

These agnosias, which are sometimes encountered in parietal lesions, imply the destruction of a receptive co-ordination centre, one of those centres where the habitual associations arise which are called forth by a given congeries of sensations to which this centre acts as representative and agent of transmission.

Among ordinary things with a symbolic value for some agreed purpose (a playing card, flag, fork, etc.) there are some, namely words, which occupy a pre-eminent place in our lives and yet have only this symbolic value. The understanding of words seems to imply the functioning of special co-ordination centres, differing according to the receptive tract.

We shall have to insist on the importance of such co-ordination centres in the mechanism of language.

The co-ordination centres, unlike the receptive centres or the incito-motor centres, are single; they are located in one hemisphere only and serve as correspondents for the receptive centres of both sides. They are generally situated in the left hemisphere, but sometimes in the right hemisphere among left-handed people. Pure word-blindness, for instance, is well-known; it is accompanied by a right hemianopsia, because the lesion that damages the co-ordination centre necessary for reading, located in the left hemisphere, also damages the optic tract of this hemisphere, passing under the cortex to reach the occipital pole. But cases are cited where visual agnosia of written words, or alexia, is accompanied by a left hemianopsia.

The existence of localized co-ordination centres does not seem any longer open to discussion; the exact determination of their position, however, may still provide matter for controversy, as we shall see later on.

4. *Incito-motor Co-ordination Centres*

Just as there may be agnosia without anæsthesia—such as word-blindness, that is to say an incapacity to read, without blindness—so there may also be an 'apraxia' without paralysis, that is to say, an incapacity to execute actions, complex habitual movements, though the power to execute voluntarily all the necessary isolated movements remains unimpaired. An individual will no longer be able to perform such habitual actions as blowing his nose or making the sign of the cross.

Such a disorder would follow lesions and wounds in the parietal lobe, and especially in the lower parietal convolution, on the left side among right-handed people, the co-ordination centre of these habitual movements being one-sided, as are the receptive co-ordination centres. This localization is, however, still somewhat doubtful—though the existence of a localization is not.[1]

If the isolated injured centre is the co-ordination centre of verbal execution, of language, we have aphasia, which is supposed to be purely motor, or aphemia, Pierre Marie's anarthria. Without autopsies, we could not hope that war lesions would enable us to fix precisely the seat of a centre—vainly conceived as a storehouse of motor images—which was located as a result of Broca's work at the foot on the third frontal, and which Pierre Marie could only place in a somewhat wide quadrilateral area, excluding Broca's centre but extending right up to it. On the whole, the anatomical controversy as such is of less importance than is generally supposed: whether the centre is found in the insula,

[1] The interruption of the communication tracts of the two hemispheres, through lesion of the corpus callosum, involves unquestionable apraxias—as well as remarkable intellectual disturbances—and induces us to think that certain parietal lesions cause disturbances of praxic co-ordination, rather by symmetrical section of the principal association paths of the co-ordination centre than by real destruction of this centre which various considerations empirically supported lead us to place in the frontal region. In particular we may cite one of Sierra's cases, where he describes a characteristic apraxia, accompanying an abscess of the sinus which compressed the frontal region and disappeared after the operation (1920). In an interesting article devoted to apraxia Roncoroni very properly points out that 'eupraxia,' which implies a complex circuit, with multiple stations, may be disturbed by lesions affecting very different points, quite apart from apraxias due to the distant reverberations of certain lesions—to the effects of diaschisis ("Le basi anatomiche dell aprassia," *Rivista sperimentale di Freniatria*, 1924, XLVIII, pp. 637-665).

that part of the cortex which is folded back under the fissure of Sylvius, continuing the area of the third frontal to the very edge of the fissure, or in another point of the quadrilateral, matters very little in a general way.

The controversy, however, gave rise to the view that there would be no further localization, since Broca's centre had been proved a failure. Feeling ran high where beliefs and convictions were involved such as science should always mistrust in spite of their evident respectability, and this led to an over-speedy triumph and to some misunderstanding.

The war was responsible for cases of aphemia resulting from lesions in the Broca-Marie area; and it can safely be affirmed that the co-ordination centre necessary to verbal execution is to be found in this area.

As for the general conception of the mechanism of language and aphasia, it is outside this particular controversy. We shall consider it again later as a whole.

5. *The Problem of Intellectual Centres*

Reference is often made to 'association centres,' but this term covers in a general way such parts of the brain as are not occupied by 'projection' centres, or by receptive or sensori-motor centres—which is a negative specification. In reality it is the brain as a whole which is the centre of association, and the association is the very raison d'être of the nervous system as a whole.

But it has sometimes been held that there are intellectual centres, which constitute the seat of well-defined mental functions; and an imaginary anatomy has been used in these schematic constructions. There have been attempts to localize the intelligence, the higher psychic states, etc.; and the highest functions have generally been assigned to the frontal lobe, because of its great development in man.

But after what we have said of the functioning of

the cerebral system, the impossibility of ever localizing actual entities, like attention, memory,[1] and intelligence will be realized. We do not localize in the parts of a machine qualities such as its speed, its output, its regular or silent working,[2] etc. In particular, the intelligence is a value-judgment which we pass on the functioning of a cerebral machine. But what we are judging is the total functioning in its entirety, from a certain point of view; and the point of view, though the same term *intelligence* is used, often varies from one judgment to another.

Suppress all the receiving, co-ordinating and activating centres and you suppress the functioning of the machine; suppress a few of these centres and you get a disturbance which though not unimportant (anæsthesia, functional paralysis, asymbolia, and apraxia) does not completely prevent the system from working.

Theoretically, so long as a receptive centre remains, a certain functioning is still possible, doubtless very much reduced if there is not at least one symbolic co-ordination centre left.[3] But it is obvious that as between different individuals the same defect can have

[1] The centre of memory is often conceived as a storehouse of images. But there are no images apart from sensation; and just as the atom of traditional chemistry is now a system of electrons, so the image, the static entity of traditional psychology, should also be resolved into a dynamic system, a process of sensory evocation.

[2] Larguier des Bancels justly observes that the "centres have long lent support to mere abstractions," and that faculties are still being localized, "complex functions whose elements alone can be localized in the proper sense of this word." (*Introduction à la Psychologie. L'Instinct et l'Émotion*, 1921, p. 74).

[3] A man blinded by complete bilateral cortical destruction of the occipital centres no longer has visual images of any kind, and cannot even represent to himself the nature of vision. This is true in spite of the contrary assertions of Monakow, and we shall return to the matter again. Hence there can be no sort of visual thought; the suppression of all the receptive areas—including the kinæsthetic—would be incompatible with thought in any form. But it is quite clear that peripheral suppression of all sensibility would not have the same result, at any rate if it occurred only after a certain experience of life; there would remain, in fact, possibilities of internal evocation of sensations and the employment of images. An incito-associative capacity would remain through mnemonic persistence.

very different consequences; an orator who thinks aloud, a painter whose visual imagination represents his habitual form of mental activity, a musician who hears harmonies repeated or created within him, will not be equally affected by a lesion which attacks either the linguistic co-ordination centres or the visual centres or the auditory centres or the association bundles in the neighbourhood of these centres.

In particular—if we use the word intelligence as a synonym for mental activity, as is often done—we must differentiate between the primitive forms of sensory intelligence, with their ill-developed symbolism beyond which backward children cannot advance, as Binet well observed, and the forms of verbal intelligence created by social education, abstract and conceptual forms. Complete sensory aphasia will notably diminish mental activity in one of these forms of intelligence, and will have no very marked effect on sensory intelligence.

We are thus able to appreciate why lesions have been described sometimes as having the most serious consequences, sometimes as having no appreciable effect; and this has led certain people to think, or rather to justify their belief, that the brain plays only an accidental and secondary rôle in mental activity, and that every cerebral area is equivalent to every other.

This view claims to find justification in certain celebrated accounts, often grossly exaggerated, of cases where the brain is said to have been almost completely removed with no effect on mental activity.[1] It had already been put forward before the war, in a note by Robinson to the Académie des Sciences;[2] and more

[1] We have here a new manifestation of an old movement against the conception of cerebral localization. It was originally related directly to the work of Goltz, who cited cases of considerable loss of substance, revealed by autopsy, where nothing during the life of the individual thus cerebrally deficient would have suggested such serious lesions.

[2] R. Robinson, "Les localisations physiologiques de l'encéphale en contraste avec les destructions étendues de cet organe," *C. R. Ac. des Sc.*, 1913, Vol. CLVII, p. 1463. The case is that of a man of 62, wounded in

especially during the war it was voiced in a series of papers by Guépin on cerebral surgery:[1] the excision of cerebral lesions is said to have led to the removal of a third of the left hemisphere (occipital area) of a wounded soldier who afterwards showed no signs either of diminished intelligence or of sensori-motor disturbance. But what can be deduced from an observation in which there was no accurate examination to prove what had been removed? On this occasion there was an abscess, and in such cases pus is often mistaken for cerebral matter—but the evacuated leucocytes do not act as neurones.

I had the opportunity of examining the brain of a war case which I had studied, where there was an operation for a deep abscess in the frontal region. The surgeon, after cleaning out the abscess, had found a cavity the size of a fist. Not only were there psychical disturbances which might have passed unnoticed in rapid examination, but the loss of cerebral substance was in reality insignificant. After cleaning out the pus which had formed the cavity, not so much by destruction as by pushing matter aside, the tissues had taken their place again and there was very little injury apart from a small nuclear scar. But the surgeon had honestly supposed that a great part of the hemisphere had been destroyed.

This shows what reservations are necessary in dealing with these sensational observations, especially when they are being treated sensationally, without either a satisfactory mental examination or a really careful

the head, where the autopsy revealed that all the lobes were "very considerably mortified." According to the preliminary investigation, "his intelligence was slightly affected and his memory somewhat impaired. The patient did not suffer in any way; he was content and happy. His speech was a little disturbed but this might have been due to lack of teeth" (?). The inadequacy of the anatomical examination is equalled only by the nullity of the mental examination.

[1] *Cf. C. R. Ac. des Sc.* 1915, Vol. CLX, p. 400, Vol. CLXI, p. 703, and *Le Caducée*, May 15, 1916, p. 74 (A. Guépin, "Dix cas de chirugie cérébrale").

cerebral examination—and sometimes without even the possibility of a cerebral examination.[1]

What is quite certain is that though a small and strictly limited lesion, located in certain areas, may involve well-defined and often very serious disturbances —for the receptive and incito-motor brain centres have never been excised without causing some damage— lesions much more widely extended and larger destructions may only produce effects difficult to determine.

Mental functioning, which consists in associations bringing into play various agents of the receptive stations (evocation of images) or incitor and especially co-ordinating stations, may continue even when certain association paths are interrupted and destroyed. In fact the enormous multiplicty of these tracts allows of substitution.

If the railway from Paris to Rheims through Soissons is cut, the traffic will go through Épernay; if Êpernay is also disconnected, the indirect track through Chaumont and Chalons is still available. Were we to judge only by the final outcome, we might conclude that the lines did not serve for transportation at all since a junction had been cut without any results.

The fact is that in both hemispheres there are countless connections—and they are rarely all destroyed at the same time—which ensures the indispensable communications. If the central stations, the distributive stations which represent the co-ordination centres, are not destroyed or disabled by the complete destruction of the lines in their immediate neighbourhood,[2] the

[1] These cases have been brought together by Troude, who is very much deceived as to their value, and their collective effect enables one to realize how little can be deduced from such evidence. ("Cerveau et Pensée," *Revue Scientifique*, June 26, 1920, pp. 359-363).

[2] Certain sub-cortical lesions—in spite of the effort that has been made to differentiate them—may have the same effect as destructions of the cortex and of its neurones. If all the tracts which lead to a station and away from it are destroyed, that will clearly be equivalent to the destruction of the station itself, except in respect of the possibility of regeneration and restitution from without.

functioning may be slightly hindered, but it will not be prevented.

The hindrance will not even be noticeable unless it concerns lines which usually bear a heavy traffic. It certainly will not be affected if the tracts are little used.[1] But if, for example, the tracts destroyed are those which put the visual receptive centres in communication with the rest of the cerebral apparatus, if communication of a visual order becomes more difficult, this will interfere with certain forms of thought demanding visual imagery, and the difficulty will be accentuated for individuals who rely especially on this form of thought. War pathology has confirmed the existence of cerebral areas serving more particularly for associations of a certain order, for different forms of thought.

6. *The Specialization of the Association Paths and Dynamic Localization*

The 'dumb' areas of the brain, those whose excitation or destruction is not immediately apparent as a sensory or motor disturbance, the areas which do not allow of 'projection centres' and which Flechsig regarded as 'association centres,' have naturally led to a variety of localizations on their *terræ ignotæ*. The frontal and parietal lobes extending over a tempero-parieto-occipital area, were regarded as the seat of important psychical functions.

Intelligence was placed sometimes in the anterior portion of the frontal lobes, whose development is considerable in man, and sometimes in the great parietal area. Memory was variously located, in consequence of continued amnesias observed during frontal

[1] A human brain represents innumerable possibilities of associative connections, but the majority of mankind use very few of them! Bianchi in his *Leçons sur les localisations cérébrales*, published at Naples in 1900, admitted the existence of great unoccupied areas. This is perhaps true for many specimens of humanity. For learned polyglots, however, this doubtless does not hold; slight lesions have more chance in their case of producing disturbances or apparent gaps.

lesions by Mabille and Pitres for example),[1] or occipital (Dide's occipital syndrome).[2] Personality and morality, as well as attention, seemed to be situated in the frontal convolutions.

In his essay on the interpretation of the results of autopsies or of surgical cures of mental disorders, Hollander regarded the parietal lobe as a centre of emotions affected in melancholia, and of sensory fusion; and the frontal lobe—affected in mania—as a combination of the centres of association, imagination, perception, memory, and all the higher intellectual processes, as well as the centre of voluntary control and moral, æsthetic and religious feeling.[3]

Moreover, serious lesions of the frontal region may pass unperceived, which naturally leads many writers to deny the anterior lobe of the brain any part in intellectual operations.

It is certainly absurd to look for a cerebral seat of personality, which objectively is an expression of the law of the unity of nervous functioning, and subjectively appears as a complex feeling, the result of a certain mode of mental functioning and formed under the influence of social education.[4] And how can we localize

[1] Mabille and Pitres, "Sur un cas d'amnésie de fixation post-apoplectique ayant persisté pendant vingt-trois ans," *Revue de Médecine*, 1913, XXXIII, pp. 257-279. The pre-frontal lobe was isolated in this case by a lesion which affected the long associative bundles.

[2] *Cf.* M. Dide and Ch. Pezet "Syndrome occipital," *Bull. de la Soc. clin. de Méd. mentale*, 1913, VI, pp. 279-291.

[3] Hollander, *The Mental Symptoms of Brain Disease*, London, 1910. It is of interest that after an anatomico-clinical examination of 3000 lunatics, Anglade, like Hollander, inclines to connect melancholia with a parietal disturbance and mania with a frontal lesion (*cf.* Anglade, "Les terriroires intellectuels du cerveau," *L'Encéphale*, 1921, XVI, pp. 423-437). Loeb, who attributed to the anterior brain of the dog the inhibitory function (since animals deprived of the frontal region displayed agitation and violent instincts), and to the posterior brain as a whole the inverse excitor function, had already connected these data with manic agitation, in which excessive expenditure of activity is contrasted with the exaggeration of inhibition in melancholia.

[4] *Cf.* Blondel, "La personnalité," *Journal de Psychologie*, XVII, 3, 4, 1920, p. 193 and p. 309.

intelligence, which is only the successful adaptation of all mental functioning, whether original and creative or merely assimilative? Such adaptation will give rise to an appreciation, a judgment of value, which may indeed create an idea, a concept, but can engender the entity, Intelligence, only in the same sense that our æsthetic admiration of the setting sun may be said to engender Intrinsic Beauty.[1] Are we to seek for a centre of attention when this function, though it appears under this name in the study of psychological mechanisms, is one of the most general in the whole nervous system, in the form of reinforcements and inhibitions so co-ordinated as to ensure functional unity, the unity of organic individuality? Finally, can memory be represented solely in one area of the brain, seeing that the mnemonic function makes its appearance with living substance itself, while the facilitation of a nervous tract, to which all forms of memory can be reduced, represents a basic law which is certainly not confined to the brain, though it is only in connection with associative functioning that we find this general property of the nervous system in the particular form usually known as memory?

The psychological ideas inherited from traditional systems and elaborated by a generation more interested in moral education than in scientific knowledge, notions of faculties conceived as independent entities or collections of psychical states which had only to be assigned their place in compartments of the soul or in those of the brain, do not readily lend themselves to that correlation of nervous and mental functioning which Gall made a premature attempt to establish.

But the dynamic ideas to which the experimental study of the mind has led are closely allied to the dynamic ideas imposed on the anatomists themselves by the experimental study of nervous functions.[2] Anatomy

[1] *Cf.* H. Piéron, "La Mémoire," *Revue Philosophique*, 1918, 43rd year, 9-10, pp. 240-281, and *Traité de Psychologie*.

[2] The representation of mental phenomena in the form of reactions, conditioned reflexes, Bechterew's 'psycho-reflexes,' leads to a truly physiological

can no longer confine itself to the artificial morphological peculiarities of the lobes of the brain, nor to collections of corpses embalmed by a gum fixative and examined under the microscope.[1] The superficial division into compartments which we owe to anatomists ignorant of the laws of functioning of a living nervous system, and to psychologists occupied only in collecting mental facts without even suspecting that there could be laws governing the evolution of psychical processes has led and still leads to these contradictory and absurd localizations.

But the reaction against puerile theories must not lead to an equally false conception which would only allow the brain an unimportant part in mental activity, as a reservoir of energy or an undifferentiated sub-stratum that could fulfil all its functions by intensified effort in spite of quantitative reductions, just as a small piece of lung can effect oxygenation or a single kidney can take the place of the other kidney if it disappears or is weak.[2]

schematization of cerebral localization (*cf.* W. Bechterew, "La localisation des psycho-reflexes dans l'écorce cérébrale," *Scientia*, 1916, pp. 444-457).

[1] Von Monakow, for example, introduced the idea of successive localization: a cerebral process implies the bringing into play of a group of neurones, takes place in time and may involve *points d'appui* situated at a distance.

The simplest facts of elementary physiology imply, of course, that any process whatever must take place in time. The mere admission that the neuronic layers are capable of functioning would suggest that in their functioning time must count.

But Von Monakow has also developed a concept of 'chronogenic' localization, and has introduced as factors in the process groups both differently situated and of a different age from the point of view of ontogenetic or phylogenetic evolution (*cf.* Von Monakow, *Die Lokalisation im Grosshirn*, 1914).

[2] Shepherd Ivory Franz reaches this sort of conclusion. As a result of experiments on animals he claims that even the functions of projection reappeared after a temporary disturbance and that the processes of learning remained possible with a mere remnant of the cortex, no matter where situated. But certain of his experiments on lower mammals, such as the rat, have no very general bearing, while the results of his work on monkeys, being in distinct contradiction with those of a number of other experimenters, are very doubtful: the ablations were crude and only roughly checked, and seem to have been incomplete in every case, as Von Monakow observes. (*Cf.* S. I. Franz, "Cerebral Adaptation vs. Cerebral Organology," *Psych. Bulletin*, 1917, XIV, pp, 137-140).

We shall consider at a later stage whether there is not some truth in such views. But we must not forget that in the processes due to the interaction of the cerebral neurones, there are specially important points of junction, 'synapses' which cannot be broken with impunity.

The connection of the receptive tracts with the associative area involves synapses grouped in true connecting centres, receptive and incito-associative centres, just as the associative area is connected in the incito-motor centres with the tracts of motor reaction. And in areas where the synapses are complex and varied, apart from the co-ordinating junctions, there is no doubt that the interruption of a particular tract, or the destruction of a given relay neurone involved in a process does not render impossible the definite process which normally involves this tract or this neurone. But the fact that an equivalent process occurs will generally prevent the discovery of a lacuna, which is in any case small, and which, even if there were no substitution, would clearly be very difficult to detect.

On the other hand, when the destruction affects a great number of these associative circuits, whose operation constitutes mental activity, we find many surprising modifications ;[1] but only a careful scientific examination before and after can determine the nature of the modification, and this examination has hitherto almost always been lacking.

But, rough though they may be, clinical observations on the disturbances correlated with localized lesions of the brain are not without value in providing indications

[1] There are lesions which, without touching the relays of cells, interrupt, at one point at least, all the association paths that link up the different areas of the cortex, at the level of the most superficial cortical layer, the layer of the tangential fibres. Such lesions cause serious mental disorders, the entire abolition of the mental functions, as in an interesting case reported by Marchand and Abély where a rapidly-developing sclerosis involved a parallel intellectual failure, which quickly became complete ("Démence rapide par sclérose cérébrale," *Annales médico-psychologiques*, July, 1925, pp. 185-195).

as to the nature of the principal associative circuits represented in special area.

Thus in double lesions of the occipital lobe, not necessarily affecting the receptive centres, visual thought is generally affected: the capacity for orientation and self-direction, which in most individuals demand visual schemata, is lost or very much diminished.

In the left temporal parietal region verbal thought is affected, and major lesions which disrupt the whole unity of the associative circuits may involve aphasias with considerable diminution of intellectual power; for this, in modern social life, implies the use of language, the essential instrument of 'symbolic thought.'

Various writers are in close agreement in recording that disorders of character predominate in the frontal region;[1] there is generally aboulia and apathy, but also impulsiveness and irritability, the power of inhibition being diminished, which is in agreement with Fano's experiments on monkeys;[2] a taste for childish play and a 'roguish' character sometimes appear.

In experiments in extirpation of the frontal lobes of the monkey, Bianchi[3] observed incoherence of conduct, loss of initiative and manifestations attributed to the higher sentiments (gratitude, jealously, sociability, etc.)[4]

[1] *Cf.* in particular for war lesions, Ch. Chatelin, *Les blessures du cerveau*, 1918 [E.T. 1918], and W. Poppelreuter, *Die psychischen Schädigungen durch Kopfschuss im Kriege*, Vol. II, 1917; also a good general survey by Kurt Goldstein ("Die Funktionen des Frontallappens," *Medizinische Klinik*, 1923, XXIX, Nos. 28 and 29).

[2] Fano, "Contributo alla localizzazione sur-corticale dei poteri inhibitori," *Atti della R. Ac. dei Lincei*, 1895, p. 292. *Cf.* also Fano, "Inhibition et volonte," *Rev. gén. des Sciences*, Oct. 30th, 1920, p. 649.

[3] Bianchi, *La Mécanique du cerveau* (French translation, Paris, 1921; English translation, *The Mechanism of the Brain*, Edinburgh, 1922).

[4] Loss of initiative was shown, for example, in the experiments of Affanassiev on a dog deprived of the pre-frontal area, which would eat food wrapped in paper without undoing the paper as does a normal animal. But in this case we may also regard the phenomenon as due to an insufficient inhibition of impulses which is seen very clearly in another observation by the same author: a dog whose pre-frontal lobes had been removed went and seized a lump of sugar behind a lighted match—which a normal dog would avoid (Bechterew,

This does not imply that the will, the moral sense or the higher emotions are located there ;[1] we must first be sure of their existence. But it may indicate that the affective life, the play of tendencies, involves the intervention of frontal synapses. We shall endeavour later to outline a possible view of the rôle of the affective life in mental behaviour, and of the participation of the various levels of the nervous system in this life.

In any case, though frontal injuries may be shown by affective modifications without true intellectual

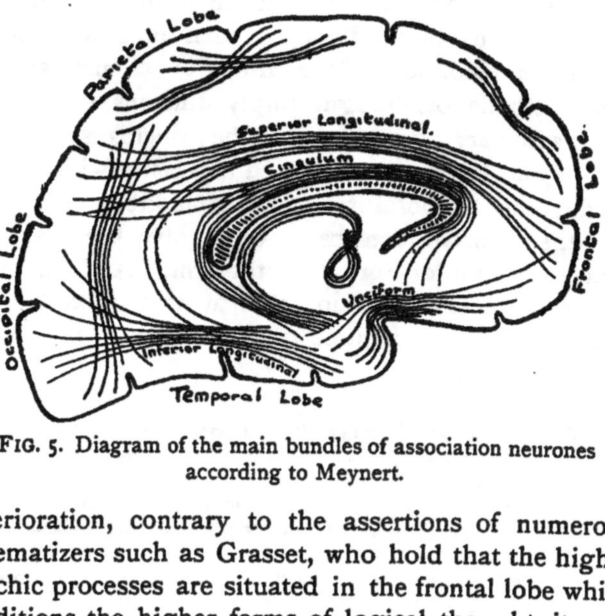

FIG. 5. Diagram of the main bundles of association neurones according to Meynert.

deterioration, contrary to the assertions of numerous schematizers such as Grasset, who hold that the higher psychic processes are situated in the frontal lobe which conditions the higher forms of logical thought, it may

"Studium der Funktionen der Prefrontal und anderer Gebiete der Hirnrinde vermittelst der associativo-motorischen Reflexe," *Archives suisses de Neurologie*, 1923, XIII, pp. 61-76).

[1] William Browning, after an analysis of eleven cases of cranial traumata followed by a serious deterioration of moral conduct without intellectual weakening, placed the 'moral centre' without hesitation in the right frontal lobe, the lesion of the first frontal convolution involving irritability, violence, and the loss of the inhibitory power, and that of the second and third frontal convolutions, the loss of the 'moral sense,' and the complete disappearance of the feelings of shame, fear, of the command of duty, or of simple cleanliness (*Medical Record*, June 18th and 25th, 1921).

be noted that certain injuries, which doubtless destroy privileged synapses, may reappear as definite disturbances of activity, as praxic disorders. Such is the syndrome of disorientation in space, of which Pierre Marie and Béhague[1] have given interesting examples.

The association paths which predominate in the various cerebral areas seem to depend strictly on the nearest receptive or incito-motor centres, and the corresponding co-ordination areas—which is easily comprehensible. The various forms of thought, the processes of association, may be carried on with a dominant sensory nucleus that differs for each individual, and in a given individual, according to circumstances. These methods of thought imply different functional circuits with varying positions for the principal synapses. The occipital tracts are concerned especially with visual thought, the temporal tracts with auditory thought, while the frontal tracts seem to involve the play of affective and motor forms of thought. And parietal tracts, in the case of a blind and deaf person like Helen Keller can certainly assume predominance in the form of tactile thought.[2]

[1] *Cf.* Pierre Marie and Béhague, " Syndrome de désorientation dans l'espace consécutif aux plaies profondes du lobe frontal," *Revue Neurologique*, 1919, XXVI, pp. 3-14. The syndrome would arise from an interruption of the association bundles, which link the anterior frontal area with other cerebral areas. According to the data provided it would seem to be a question of a disorder of conduct, a praxic disorder. " It is impossible for me to distinguish in the dark," said one of the wounded patients, " whether I am turning to the right or the left." But he knew the direction to follow and could indicate it. Spatial representation (at least through visual schemata) is possible, contrary to what we find in cases of disorientation through occipital lesion; but motor activity becomes impossible. In fact, we have here a disturbance of kinesthetic thought while spatial visual thought remains perfectly correct. A fresh and very characteristic account of this syndrome has been given more recently by Pierre Marie, Bouttier and Van Bogaert (" Un cas de tumeur préfrontale droite," *Revue Neurologique*, 1924, XXXI (II), pp. 209-221).

[2] No doubt the forms of thought of various animals—however rudimentary they may appear, especially owing to their lack of social education by language—will have very different sensory bases; in the case of the dog, thought must clearly be mainly olfactory.

It is round the co-ordination centres of verbal symbolism which are located in a single hemisphere, that the tracts of abstract thought which operate through language and the concept—the symbol of a symbol—naturally radiate. These tracts extend particularly from the posterior part of the parietal and temporal lobes to the level of the angular gyrus as far as the foot of the frontal convolutions, from the area of receptive co-ordination to that of executive co-ordination.

7. *General Disturbances of Cerebral Function—Nervous 'Tension'*

In cerebral lesions there are functional disturbances which may appear whatever the seat of the lesion, but which, in virtue of a *post hoc ergo propter hoc* have been regarded as symptomatic of injury to all the cerebral areas in succession.

Thus it is with the weakening of the memory, or, more accurately, diminution of the power of fixing memories on the one hand and of evoking old memories on the other; and similarly with the lowering of the capacity of attention and mental effort, from the double standpoint of intensity and duration (rapid fatigue).

The phenomena of continous amnesia, the complete absence of mnemonic registration, have been noted in cases of occipital, parietal and frontal lesions. Sluggishness, difficulty of recall—which is only a form of sluggishness, of difficulty in associative processes and in intellectual operations generally—is found constantly in cerebral injuries And fatigability of attention, inability to make an intense and sustained effort, goes along with it.

Grasset proposed the term 'atopical' symptoms for disorders observed in patients suffering from cerebral lesions, independently of the seat of the lesion, as opposed to symptoms of localization.[1] He meant by

[1] *Cf. Montpellier Médical*, 1916, XXXIX, 1.

this, however, the signs of a cerebral lesion. But though these wounds are usually followed by general symptoms, among which are the psychical disorders just mentioned and called by Pierre Marie 'subjective' symptoms, this is not necessarily the case. They may appear without any cerebral injury, as a result of cranial traumata, which are even more intense when the shock is not complicated by craniotomy; or as a result of general traumata such as shock due to violent disturbances of air-pressure produced by bursting shells.[1]

Such symptoms are not connected, as Grasset's expression suggests, with a limited destruction of the brain wherever this may occur, but with a disturbance of cellular activity as a whole by disturbance of neuronic metabolism.[2]

These effects are analogous to those that may be produced by a generalized toxic action, an insufficiency of oxygen due to asphyxiation or compression (in the course of cerebral tumours for example), or as a result of generalized circulatory disorders. In organic lesions of the brain, these general functional disorders naturally tend to vary not with the seat but with the nature and reverberation of the lesion.

Here we must introduce an idea that is quantitative rather than qualitative. Cerebral activity, in the course of intellectual process, implies an expenditure of nervous energy through consumption of the reserves stored up in the cells and replenished by the nutritive contribution or the mobilization of reserves situated in other organs.

If the reserves be impoverished and poorly replenished, if the chemical process of consumption of reserves be

[1] Disorders of memory and of attention are elements of the 'concussion syndrome' which A. Mairet and the author were among the first to distinguish in the first months of the war (*Cf.* "Le syndrome commotionnel dans les traumatismes de guerre," *Bulletin de l'Académie de Médecine*, June 1st, 15th and 22nd, 1915).

[2] *Cf.* A. Mairet and H. Piéron, "De la différenciation des symptômes commotionnels et des symptômes atopiques dans les traumatismes cranio-cérébraux," *Montpellier Médical*, 1916, XXXIX, 6.

interfered with, cerebral activity will become difficult and irregular—will be diminished, retarded and contracted. The most difficult processes, these demanding a high degree of attention, an augmented 'nervous tension' with numerous and intense reinforcements and inhibitions, will be most affected. The most automatic circuits, those which are the most isolated and the most easily brought into play, along well-worn paths where the resistance of the synapses is weakest, will continue —and the more readily in that they are inhibited with greater difficulty.

Functional disturbances will occur in a constant order because it will be the order of the increasing difficulty of the process involved.

Whatever area of the brain remains at work when others are destroyed, the same characteristic disturbances of function will appear.[1] Processes of high tension will be the first to be abolished,[2] the most automatic being the most tenacious.

Now the amount of potential energy accumulated in the cerebral cells as a whole will have its influence, so that localized destructions, by diminishing the total reserve, may thereby, quite apart from a whole repercussion on metabolism, cause a diminution of nervous tension when the cerebral machine is functioning to the full.

That this is not impossible is no doubt due not to the influence of potential reserves, but to the fact that complex operations bring into play various elements in

[1] It may happen that the functional disturbance does not extend to the entire cerebral system, but remains limited to one area which is compressed, insufficiently irrigated, and in more direct contact with a toxic agent, etc.; in the area which is not destroyed, there will be a selective functional diminution with a local predominance in relation to the seat of this partial injury and a hierarchic predominance in relation to the intensity of the injury.

[2] The idea of nervous 'tension' is closely related to that of psychological 'tension,' used by Pierre Janet in his acute analysis of the pathological processes of the mind. Janet, however, gives 'tension' a special sense, differentiating it from 'quantity' of energy, so that the two concepts cannot be equated forthwith.

all parts of the brain, and that the lacunæ, though they do not hinder the process itself, which is polymorphous and is doubtless never repeated in an absolutely identical fashion, can yet diminish the total quantity of nervous energy expended in the course of its accomplishment. This energy is translated into actions of reinforcement or inhibition at a distance, and appears in the direction of thought and the regulation of conduct.

But if there is such an influence, it is probably not very considerable. And the growth of the volume of the brain with the intellectual level in the evolution of the vertebrates cannot be regarded as simply correlative to the increase of potential energy accumulated where the neurones are densest.

It is the increasing multiplicity of possible association circuits which brings about the biological enrichment of thought,[1] and makes possible the social gain secured by language and the play of collective symbolic thought.

[1] Where there is equality of psychical organization, animals of allied species have an encephalon which increases with the surface of the body (sensory and motor surface), and especially with the number of sensory impulses. The size of the retina plays a considerable part in the development of the brain, among birds and fishes, for example. The law of proportions established by Dubois, the Dutch anthropologist, and verified and interpreted by Lapicque, allows us to envisage the marginal case where the part of the encephalon representing the bodily surface, the projection, receptive or motor, might be at one with the surface of the body in the same way for all animal species. But in reality there is a fixed residue, which does not vary with the bodily surface to which the brain would be reduced if the areas of projection diminished with the body, and whose size increases in the various groups of species with their mental level, reaching its maximum in the case of man, and followed at a distance by the elephants and the anthropoid apes. This independent residue (Lapicque's coefficient *c*) is the associative part of the brain, proportionally large in very small species like the humming birds (where the weight of the brain is far greater than that of man in comparison with the weight of the body), and proportionally negligible in huge species like the whale (where the absolute weight of the brain implied by the representation of enormous surfaces is much greater than that of man). A clear outline of these very interesting data may be found in Larguier des Bancels' *Introduction à la Psychologie*, 1921, pp. 116-125, "L'intelligence et le cerveau," and particularly in a critical survey by Lapicque himself, where much light is thrown on the disturbing influences and where the law is analysed and interpreted ("Le poids du cerveau et l'intelligence," *Journal de Psychologie*, 1922, XIX, pp. 5-23).

Part II

THE RECEPTIVE AND INCITO-MOTOR FUNCTIONS

(The elementary modes of sensori-motor thought)

Chapter I

MOTOR INCITATION

By local stimulation at certain points on the cerebral cortex, if the necessary precautions are taken to avoid diffusion,[1] we obtain in the higher mammals, such as dogs, cats and monkeys, movements of well-determined groups of muscles. We thus get the clearest idea of localization, for we can control the cause and at the same time witness the visible objective effect. There are 'motor centres'[2] whose topography might be determined with complete accuracy for every species.

[1] Very weak electrical stimulation has been chiefly used; a sufficiently strong and prolonged stimulus will be followed by motor reactions in very varied regions even in the case of an anæsthetized animal. This may result from a diffusion of the stimulus; or it may bring into play an associative circuit with a motor reactive termination. There are, then, certain favoured responses; this fact is sometimes very marked, as in the case of movements of the eyes produced by a definite occipital stimulus in the chimpanzee, according to Sherrington's experiments (*cf.* J. D. Stout, "On the Motor Functions of the Cerebral Cortex of the Cat," *Psychobiology*, 1917, I, pp. 177-229).

[2] We no longer need to recall that an incitation proceeds from these centres which will release the directly efficacious excitation of the motor neurones of the spinal cord. When we stimulate the cerebral centres with induction shocks, the currents of action of the muscle have a frequency independent of that of the shocks, while the frequency remains the same—up to about a hundred per second—when the irritation bears on the spinal cord (*cf.* P. Hoffmann, "Ueber die Innervation des Muskels bei Groszhirnreizung," *Arch. für Physiologie*, 1910, supp. 3, pp. 223-249).

It would seem that in this field physiological experiments afford the best opportunity of extending to man the general conclusions obtained from the species most akin to him, the more so in that we have been able to apply the same method to man himself during surgical operations.[1]

This method has allowed us to separate off in the Rolandic region, which is regarded as sensitivo-motor, an area limited to the ascending frontal convolution, with an exclusively motor character, parallel to the ascending parietal behind the fissure of Rolando, which is exclusively sensory; the functional difference corresponding to an entirely different structure.[2]

On the pre-Rolandic convolution we find an arrangement, analogous in the monkey and in man, by which different parts of the body, on opposite sides, are represented in layers on each hemisphere in reverse order: above, across the convex surface of the hemisphere, are the motor centres of the lower limb; below, the trunk (at any rate in the case of the chimpanzee) occupying very little space; below that again, the arm, the forearm and the hand, with a greatly enlarged projection for the movements of the fingers; finally at the base of the convolution, the centres of the muscles of the face, the jaws, and the larynx.

The area occupied by the incito-motor surfaces is by no means proportional to the size or number of the muscles of the body. Some of the musculature of the

[1] The principal researches on man are due to Krause (*Chirurgie des Gehirns und Rückenmarcks*, 1911), on the anthropoid ape to Grünbaum and Sherrington ("Observations on the Physiology of the Cerebral Cortex," *Proc. Royal Soc.*, 1901, LXIX, p. 206, 1903, LXXII, p. 152).

[2] In the motor area, or at least in the greater part of this area, we find a layer of giant pyramidal cells, called the cells of Betz, which seem to be the elements directly in connection—through their axonic prolongations which constitute the pyramidal bundle—with the medullary motor neurones. From a systematic examination of numerous brains of the insane, Ladame concluded that motor disturbances are always accompanied by changes in Betz' cells, while injury to these cells is always accompanied by motor disturbances (*Cf. Encéphale*, 1911, VI, pp. 532-535).

trunk cannot even be detected in the human brain, while the thumb and the index finger alone occupy a considerable cortical surface, almost as large as the entire leg.[1] The musculature of the bucco-laryngeal region has also a very extensive projection. The complexity of the possible movements is here a factor of the first importance, and so too is their psychical value.

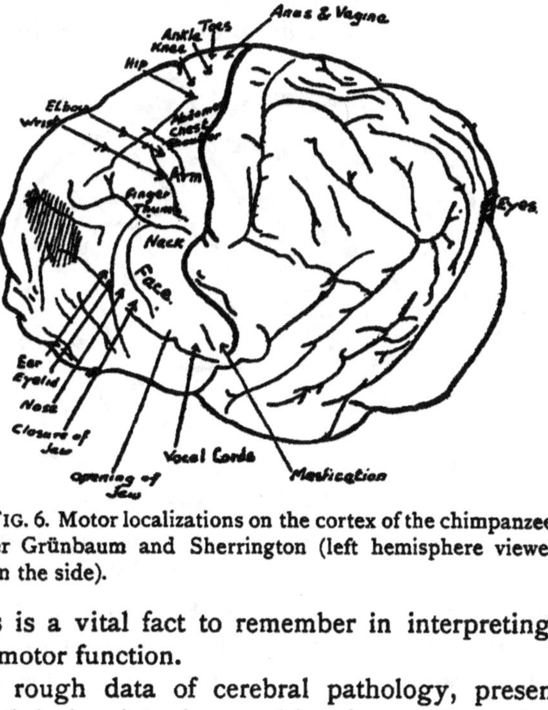

FIG. 6. Motor localizations on the cortex of the chimpanzee, after Grünbaum and Sherrington (left hemisphere viewed from the side).

This is a vital fact to remember in interpreting the incito-motor function.

The rough data of cerebral pathology, presenting left or right hemiplegias resulting from ordinary lesions in the right or left hemisphere (compressions through

[1] In the various species there is a connection between the development of the limbs and the incito-motor surfaces of the pre-Rolandic precentral cortex, and also between this development and that of the anterior horns of the spinal cord, where the motor neurones are situated. Thus the gibbon, which has extraordinarily well-developed front limbs, has a more extensive excito-motor surface than the orang or the chimpanzee, and a wider extension of the giant cells of Betz (*Cf.* F. W. Mott, E. Schuster, C. S. Sherrington, "Motor Localization in the Brain of the Gibbon correlated with an Histological Examination," *Folia Neuro-Biologica*, 1911, V, pp. 699-707).

hæmorrhage, softening due to occlusion of the nutrient artery, etc.), were insufficient to confirm the exact localization of direct excitation. Nevertheless, crural monoplegias were noted—the hemiplegia being confined to the lower limb—coincident with lesions of the upper Rolandic region ; and brachial monoplegias—the upper limb alone being affected—resulting from lower lesions.

But the war lesions, sometimes limited to very small areas pierced by a projectile, provided interesting con-

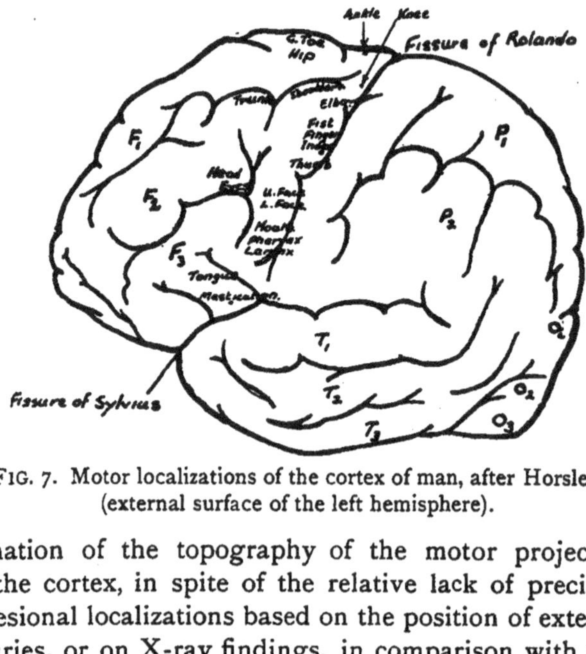

FIG. 7. Motor localizations of the cortex of man, after Horsley (external surface of the left hemisphere).

firmation of the topography of the motor projection of the cortex, in spite of the relative lack of precision in lesional localizations based on the position of external injuries, or on X-ray findings, in comparison with that attainable by direct examination.

In fact numerous cases have been observed in which motor disturbances after wounds in the Rolandic region were confined to a few muscular groups, to the hand alone, to a few fingers, or even to one finger only, the middle finger, for example.[1]

[1] Multiple wounds, such as those due to fragments of bursting shell, sometimes gave rise to various disturbances, each strictly limited ; or a wound covering the motor representation of the hand and the face might produce a limited

But there are two types of limitation in motor disturbances. One arises from the fact that unless the functional trouble is generalized but incomplete the most delicate movements are the most susceptible. Thus it is the hand which is first affected by relatively diffuse incomplete lesions or reverberations at a distance from the original lesions. The other is due to a limited partial destruction, and may affect any movements whatever, sometimes those of the shoulder; but the movements of certain fingers of the hand are often specially affected. The fact is that the corresponding centres are the most vulnerable, situated as they are at the level of the upper lateral portion of the skull, and widely spread in a region where wounds are not often mortal.

From the study of a number of war cases, Madame Athanassio-Bénisty[1] has mapped the positions of the affected centres, firstly for the thumb and the index finger (the 'radial' region of the hand) and secondly for the last three fingers (the 'ulnar' region). The first is below the second, as had already been suggested by direct electrical stimulation.

From the point of view of topographical localization, the data are most satisfying; but the same cannot be said of the motor significance of these localizations.

Let us see what occurs in the course of slight hemiplegia: after a blow with loss of consciousness, the patient on regaining consciousness is completely paralysed on one side; the limbs are inert and lifeless. After a certain time, movements again become possible; they lack precision and strength, though they improve with time; walking returns quickly, the arm is lifted and the hand closes. But finally a con-

paralysis in the muscular groups of the face and the fingers. Among the most curious cases reported we may cite that of Salkind (*Rivista ital. di Neuropatol. Psichiatr. ed Elettrot.* 1918, XI, p. 5-7). There was paresis of the right hypoglossal area and the left facial, and paralysis of the last two fingers of the left hand.

[1] *Les lésions de la zone rolandique par blessures de guerre*, 1918.

tracture often sets in which aggravates the impotence and makes it more complete. Sometimes, on the other hand, motor recovery is satisfactorily effected. By confining the hemiplegia in most cases to a limb or to part of a limb, war lesions have given us closely analogous tables of the evolution of motor disturbances.

Now recovery of voluntary movement, even when it remains incomplete, seems to be in direct contradiction with the incito-motor function of the centres situated on the ascending frontal, the pre-Rolandic convolution. And this contradiction suggests that the conception of associativo-motor centres should be rejected *in toto*.

Let us examine the matter more closely. The cortical centres are not directly motor; they can only act by means of the actual motor neurones which move the muscles, by entering into direct relation either with these neurones through the pyramidal tract, or with other sub-cortical relay centres, with co-ordination centres situated at intermediate levels.

The suppression of the superior centres, then, need not involve true paralysis, a complete suppression of movement, as the section of the fibres of the motor nerve or the destruction of the medullary centres would do. But at the beginning of the hemiplegia complete paralysis does occur. Where organic equilibrium is suddenly destroyed, we find serious disturbances at the level of all the stations connected with the one which is thus seriously affected. This is a case of 'diaschisis' in Monakow's sense. When the shock at a distance decreases, the functions dependent on the centres not directly affected will recommence little by little. Later, if the cortical injury has not been destructive, the function may be re-established, perhaps with limited sequelæ; or secondary degeneration and accentuation of the imbalance, due to the absence of one of the necessary elements for the general regulation of movement, may involve a hypertonia, or contracture of certain muscular groups such as that produced by extensive decerebration in the case of animals, and may accentuate the impotence. Finally the phenomèna of muscular atrophy, following this prolonged functional imbalance, may definitely abolish the power of movement.

In destructive lesions, after the effect of the shock is dissipated and before the secondary imbalances are developed, we can judge the results produced by the lesion in the area known as the motor cortex.

In the analysis of human hemiplegia, we are greatly aided by the study of experimental hemiplegia in the monkey, with its very similar evolution.[1]

Take, for example, the very careful experiments of Minkowski in isolated extirpation of the ascending frontal of the baboon.[2]

At first the paralysis of half the body is complete; then, on the second day, there are signs of active motility. Little by little, the movements of locomotion improve, at first in the upper part of the limbs, then at the extremities; but there are defective attitudes, a diminution of energy and speed, stiffness and a strong tendency to fatigue.

Moreover, under the influence of emotion movement is always facilitated. The animal succeeds in seizing food with its paretic arm, provided the other arm is kept motionless; but the movement remains unqualified; the fingers cannot produce isolated movements, prehension is only accomplished by the simultaneous closing of all fingers, and it is the mouth which takes the piece of apple or the bit of grape from the hand rather than

[1] This study has been conducted among several species of anthropoids, in particular by Sherrington (*cf.* Graham Brown and Sherrington, "Recovery after lesions of the motor cortex of the anthropoid ape," IX, Congrès int. de Physiol. in *Arch. int. de Physiol.*, 1913, XIV. p. 72. A. S. F. Leyton and C. S. Sherrington, "The Excitable Cortex of the Chimpanzee, Orang-utan and Gorilla," *Quart. J. of exp. Physiol.*, 1917, XI, pp. 135-222).

[2] "Étude sur la physiologie des circonvolutions Rolandiques et pariétales," *Archives suisses de Neurologie et de Psychiatrie*, 1917, I, pp. 389-459.

the hand which puts them into the mouth. There is a definite abolition of complex and delicate movements.[1]

In addition, the normal inhibition of certain reflexes and of various automatisms no longer occurs. Here we have one of the ordinary clinical facts of the semeiology of hemiplegia, 'syncinesias,' or associated automatic movements: when the animal turns its head to seize a piece of food with its mouth, the paretic arm bends and rises, for example. Some movements may cease to occur, but there will be others that are carried out of necessity and are no longer inhibited.

Loss of the power of inhibition and of regulation on the one hand, and of the capacity for effecting delicate and dissociated movements on the other, is characteristic of cortical hemiplegia.

Certain delicate movements still remain possible because their incito-motor centres are double, and being present in both hemispheres they easily supplement one another—the movements of the muscles of symmetrical action in the bucco-pharyngeal area and the larynx, for example. Double cortical injuries alone involve the labio-glosso-pharyngeal form of paralysis known as 'pseudo-bulbar,' because it presents some analogy with that which results from injury of the motor neurones actually situated in the bulb (Duchenne's labio-glosso-laryngeal paralysis).

The great automatic systems, such as walking which is represented in the spinal chord, and movements of

[1] Meier Muller, who made an anatomical study of the brain of a chimpanzee from which Graham Brown and Sherrington had removed the motor areas, considers that it is the technical reproduction of complex and differentiated movements which is affected in lesions of these 'pseudo-motor' areas, as the activations of movements extends over wide cortical areas ("Observations anatomo-physiologiques sur la région du bras dans l'écorce cérébrale," *Arch. suisses de Neur. et de Ps.*, 1919, V, p. 270). Certainly the reactive impulse might come from any associative circuit whatever, but the realization of these movements implies the pre-Rolandic level. It does not seem that there is a co-ordination centre at this level, as the author's account suggests. The paresis established is not a simple apraxia, a forgetting of movements once learned.

emotional expression arising in the thalamic region (the intermediate brain), can function without the cortex.

The decerebrate cats of Dusser de Barenne, though deprived of the cortex of their hemispheres, would walk, wander about, eat, lick their sides, lie down and get up, mew, pant, murmur, and defend themselves.[1]

Admitting that these functions do not occur in the same degree in the case of man without the participation of the cortex, it certainly seems that the usual motor co-ordination systems have a sub-cortical representation. After ablation of the thalamus, on the other hand, the animal enters into a 'decerebrate rigidity,' and we no longer find this complex form of movement.

We must admit, therefore, that the incito-motor centres are not confined to the cerebral cortex. It follows that the voluntary reactions resulting from an associative elaboration may be liberated by the participation of localized sub-cortical centres for unqualifed movements and automatic groups.[2] For delicate dissociated movements which demand continuous control and the assistance of any available information concerning the results of execution, the associativo-motor centres are exclusively cortical, and their topography is clearly demonstrated by experiment.[3]

[1] By a double ablation of the sensori-motor region of the median fissure we obtain behaviour very analogous to that of the decerebrate animal, as in the case of the dogs of Heger and Demoor, described as 'dements.' In fact, whatever the persistent associative activity may be, it can no longer be translated into activity, into motor reactions. (*Cf.* Heger and Demoor, "Contribution à la physiologie de l'écorce cérébrale," *IVe Congrès intern de Psychologie de Paris*, 1900, *Compte rendu*, 1901, pp. 64-75).

[2] Ocular movements, whose co-ordination centres — although their seat is not yet known precisely—are situated in the bulbo-mesencephalic region, can be provoked by the stimulation of different regions of the cortex, as Grünbaum and Sherrington have shown in the case of the chimpanzee. Reflexes such as that of ocular fixation will be provoked by the cortical sensory receptions which are in direct contact with co-ordination centres and infra-cortical incito-motor centres.

[3] Basing himself on the persistence of certain acquired motor habits in the Primates, after ablation of the incito-motor area of the cortex, Lashley concludes that we can only attribute to this area an action of facilitation, apart

In the case of groups acquired by learning, delicate movements such as speech, writing, or instrumental music, for example, the additional intervention of cortical co-ordination centres, superimposed on incito-motor centres, is necessary, and its importance will be seen when we come to study language.

Among the higher animals, and especially in man, the cortical incito-motor centre has acquired primarily an inhibitory value,[1] preventing the realization of the automatic groups released by a reflex response to a given stimulus. Certain voluntary reactions may consist less in a motor incitation proper than in the diminution—though with the preservation of a certain control—of an inhibition which checks such ready-made responses as flight or aggression, during the course of emotions provoked by a given stimulus.

In order to ensure the execution of the reactions elaborated by the higher associative activities, the cortex must obey the general law of unity of the nervous system, which ensures individuality of animal behaviour. From this fact arises the general regulative and inhibitory influence of thought, which in delicate and finely graduated movements conceives modes of reaction that are more highly differentiated and more subtle.[2] This influence, which is co-existent with the tardily developed incito-motor function rendered necessary by circumstances, is exercised by means of the great pyramidal projection bundle, without any other intermediary.

from a regulation of tonus (*cf. Archives of Neurology and Psychiatry*, 1924, XII, pp. 249-276). But the negative character of this conception is undoubtedly exaggerated.

[1] But there are also inhibitions proceeding from the sub-cortical incito-motor centres: the striate body, for example, has an important co-ordinating and inhibitory function, the study of which has been facilitated by the various nervous affections which occur where it has been injured, such as Huntingdon's chorea, *paralysis agitans*, etc., which are characterized by involuntary movements (*cf.* especially Ramsay Hunt, *Brain*, 1917, XL, p. 58.)

[2] The multiplicity of highly differentiated movements of the hand explains the very wide surface occupied by the representation of that member on the incito-motor area of the cortex.

We must not suppose, however, that if we could abstract from the nervous system as a whole a motor neurone of the pre-Rolandic cortex, a giant pyramidal Betz cell, and a direct motor neurone from the anterior horn of the spinal cord, their association would suffice to ensure normal motor functioning. There are complex influences arising at other levels which act upon the motor neurone; the thalamus, the striate body, and the cerebellum have influences of their own without which motor imbalance would follow.

Von Monakow very rightly insists on these interrelated groups which interact constantly, and he shows that in what he calls the 'kinetic melody' they are only isolated chords which can be localized in the anterior Rolandic convolution, while in order to localize the melody as a whole the intervention of the sub-cortical nuclei, the cerebellum, the pons, and the spinal cord, is necessary.

The fact remains that privileged chords arise at well-defined points of the pre-central cortex and that synapses occur there—connections of neurones—which control the play of certain definite movements,[1] all the rest of the system being in equilibrium and in apparent repose. We localize in the mechanism the apparatus for effecting certain pre-determined shunting operation.[2]

[1] Vulpian regarded the psycho-motor centre as a cross-road, from a truly physiological standpoint; but the static thought of the localizing anatomists no longer took into account the complexity of the functional circuits, without which we could not conceive of activity in the nervous system.

[2] According to Lashley, the connections of the cortical neurones with the groups of motor neurones in physiologically variable. He found that from one day to another the electrical stimulation of the same point of the cortex provoked different movements ("Temporal Variation in the Function of the Gyrus Precentralis in Primates," *American Journal of Physiology*, 1923, LXV, pp. 585-602). But the exact localization of electrical excitation is liable to variable diffusion and is too uncertain to allow us to accept this conclusion as the basis of the facts at present available.

CHAPTER II

SENSORY RECEPTION

THE functioning of the cortical receptive apparatus which corresponds to all the diffuse sensations of the organism, all, that is to say, which are not exclusively concentrated, like sight, hearing, taste or smell, on limited surfaces—and in proportion as they approach the cortex—involves many complex problems. We will approach these problems in the order of increasing difficulty, dealing first with the topography of cortical reception in its relation to the topography of the body, then with the relations of the various types of sensation, and finally with perception, before considering the significance of the receptive functions of the cortex from the standpoint of sensori-motor activity in general.

1. *Receptive Topography of the Diffuse Sensations of the Organism*

The stimulation in the cortex of a terminal reception of sensory excitation cannot, when it enters the associative area, be represented in a form that is immediately apparent, like the excitation of the reactive centres on leaving this area. We are obliged to have recourse indirectly to reactions which indicate the efficacy of the excitation. In the case of an animal, we cannot procure a satisfactory analysis during anæsthetic sleep with localized electrical stimulation. The use of a limited chemical excitation, touching one point of the cortex with a tampon soaked in a weak coloured solution or strychnine (Dusser de Barenne) or placing a cylinder of blotting paper soaked in such a solution at the level of a certain surface (Amantea), allows us to produce a lasting stimulation, a localized hyperæsthesia. This is translated in the behaviour of the animal by spontaneous gestures (licking and scratching), and by violent reactions to light pressures applied at the level of the region of the hyper-æsthetized body, and in addition by sensori-motor associative reverberations through reaction at a distance on association centres.[1]

These experiments have revealed a sensory cortical area, distinct from the incito-motor area but very close to it, upon which the body is represented, again inversely, so that the sensory or motor projection of the same region or of the same part of a limb is found at the same level.

In man, direct study of the cortical stimulation of the sensory area has rarely been possible. None the less, evidence of the first importance has been furnished by the American neurophysiologist and surgeon, Harvey Cushing.[2]

Cushing, by unipolar faradization, with more than fifty anæsthetized patients, confirmed the conclusions of the researches on the ape by Sherrington and Grunbaum as to the existence of motor points only in front

[1] *Cf.* Amantea, "Sur les rapports entre les centres corticaux de la circonvolution sigmoïde et la sensibilité cutanée chez le chien," *Arch. ital. de Biologie*, 1915, LXII, pp. 143-148, and "Sur les rapports topographiques entre l'écorce cérébrale et la sensibilité cutanée chez le chien," *Archives intern. de Physiologie*, 1921, XVIII, pp. 474-483: also J. G. Dusser de Barenne, "Récherches expérimentales sur la localisation de la sensibilité dans l'écorce du cerveau," *Arch. neerl. de Physiol.*, I, pp. 15-26. In Dusser de Barenne's experiments on the cat, the excitation of certain areas reacted on the sensibility of the two sides of the body, probably through nervous transmission of the hyperæsthetizing stimulation from one hemisphere to the other. The same phenomena have also been noted in the latest researches on the monkey (J. G. Dusser de Barenne, "Experimental Researches on Sensory Localization in the Cerebral Cortex of the Monkey," *Proc. Royal Soc.*, 1924, B. 96, pp. 272-291).

[2] Harvey Cushing, *loc. cit.* "A Note upon the Faradic Stimulation of the Postcentral Gyrus in Conscious Patients," *Brain*, XXXII, 1909, pp. 44-53.

of the Rolandic fissure. In addition to this he made two comparative attempts at pre- and post-Rolandic stimulation with two subjects who were awake and conscious. In both cases, after the usual osteoplastic craniotomy under general anæsthesia, cortical stimulation was subsequently possible without any anæsthesia.

The first case was that of a boy of fifteen, who suffered from sensory convulsions originating in the right hand and extending to the arm and face. The exposure of the Rolandic region revealed nothing, either on the surface or at a depth, after a parietal incision parallel to the fissure. Pre-Rolandic excitation along the fissure elicited, in descending order, flexion of the elbow, flexion and extension of the fingers, opposition of the thumb, and various movements in the region of the face. Posterior to the central fissure, stimulation produced finger-sensations of a complex nature, analogous to those preceding an attack; and a little lower down vague and diffused sensations of warmth in the arm, with the impression of choking.

The second case dealt with a man of 44, suffering from attacks of Jacksonian epilepsy, often limited to the right hand, with an aura characterized by a sensation like an electric shock running between the little and ring fingers. A high lesion was discovered, beneath which post-Rolandic excitation gave sensations of 'touching' or 'stroking' on the fingers or on the hand, according to the points stimulated; sensations were located in the index finger for an excitation opposite the motor points governing the flexion of the thumb.

In the case of Cushing's first patient, the operation constituted a true physiological experiment in localized extirpation.

In the course of the operation an incision had been made, with local ligature of the vessels, along the ascending parietal, parallel to the fissure of Rolando, in the region where electrical stimulation had produced sensations at the level of the little finger. This was done because a twitching of the little finger had occurred during the seizures. In consequence of this strictly localized minimal incision, sensory disturbances were noted in the two last fingers and the ulnar part of the hand in the form of thermal hypo-algesia and hypoæsthesia with loss of the sense of posture in the little finger.

Disturbances limited to half the hand, either the radial side (that of the thumb), or the ulnar side, were observed with care fairly frequently during the war in connection with minor lesions; and this fact caused some surprise, since it was supposed that the cortical representation of the limbs must be strictly segmental, the fingers being all juxtaposed at the same level of the ascending parietal.[1] In reality the motor points sufficed to show that the thumb and index finger are close together at a lower level than the last fingers. The functional grouping may, in a parallel manner, be more strictly responsible for the sensory projection of the internal and external surfaces of the limbs.

The hypothesis had been put forward, as early as 1906, by Russel and Horsley,[2] who, adopting the terminology of Ross and Paterson, were surprised to find that there was for each limb a 'pre-axial' half (the radial half, for the hand, innervated by the higher segments of the spinal cord viz. the fifth to the seventh cervical), and a 'post-axial' half (the ulnar half, for the hand, supplied by the lower segments, the eighth cervical and the fifth and second dorsal), with distinct

[1] This cortical segmental localization is opposed to the topography of root areas; the somatic areas are innervated by fibres which are grouped in the posterior roots of each medullary segment, cervical, dorsal and lumbar; the grouping of the fibres corresponds to re-divisions of very irregular form; and along the limbs superimposed roots innervate longitudinal parallel bands. Consequently a disturbance limited longitudinally and not transversely suggests the idea of a topography of root areas characteristic of the localization in the spinal cord.

[2] C. K. Russel and V. Horsley, "Note on Apparent Re-representation in the Cerebral Cortex of the Type of Sensory Representation as it exists in the Spinal Cord," *Brain*, XXIX, I, 1906, pp. 137-152.

projection from the axis of the limb (the central line, innervated by the eighth cervical). These authors noted that tactile hypo-æsthesias and 'atopognosias' (disturbances of localization) may behave in an altogether different way in the pre-axial and post-axial regions; and they concluded that there was something like an echo of spinal representation in the cortex, where a very distinct projection of the two halves of the limb occurs. The mid-axial line, which is differentiated, serves as a landmark from the point of view of movement.[1]

The vaguer idea of a double representation, longitudinal and transverse, had been formulated by Calligaris, who made a collection of cases of cerebral anæsthesia "of a longitudinal type," in 1910.[2]

It must certainly not be supposed that the entire surface of one side of the body is represented with its exact form in reverse order on the post-Rolandic area of the opposite hemisphere. The peripheral receptor neurones become associated with the neurones of an incito-associative function at the level of the cortex, which are almost in one-to-one correspondence with them; but the functional relationship causes congeries of neurones to be grouped very close to one another, which facilitates their interaction, and the size of the representation is connected not with the size of the peripheral receptive surface but with the density of the primary neurones. This explains the fact that the hand occupies a very important place in the cortical receptive

[1] The first observation dealing with the different behaviour of cortical origin, of the pre-axial and post-axial halves of the limbs, in which Horsley collaborated, dates from 1894, and concerns a case in which there was a transfer in the localization from one half of the limb to the other and vice versa (T. Grainger Stewart, "On a Case of Perverted Localization of Sensation or Allachæsthesia," *British Medical Journal*, January 6th, 1894, pp. 1-4).

[2] *Cf.* G. Calligaris, "Disturbi della sensibilita di origine cerebrale a tipe radicolare," *Rivista di Patologia*, 1910, 7; "L'Anesthésie cérébrale de type longitudinal," *Revue Neurologique*, 1920, XXVII, pp. 1073-1083. *Cf.* also Bergmark, "Cerebral Monoplegia, with Special Reference to Sensation and to Spastic Phenomena," *Brain*, 1910, XXXVII, pp. 342-477.

area, since distinct sensory elements corresponding to the cutaneous surface are very numerous,[1] and the kinæsthetic sensibility of various articulations also plays its part.

Though not complete in detail, the main lines of the receptive map of the sensory cortex are thus known. We know by the hemianæsthesias which generally—but not always, especially in a lasting form—accompany motor hemiplegias, and which can also, though more rarely, occur alone, that the cortical lesion involves sensory defects. We must determine the nature of these defects either in a complete half of the body[2] or in one part only, particularly in one limb (brachial or crural sensory monoplegia), and sometimes in a segment of a limb, usually therefore at its extremity. For the extremity, being more extended, is more vulnerable, and since it allows the most delicate and elaborate, and consequently the most vulnerable, forms of sensi-

[1] According to 'Flechsig's law,' the extent of the surface of a sensory area varies with the surface of the section of the corresponding peripheral nerves, that is to say with the number of the fibres, or with the number of the neurones, whose prolongations constitute the trunk of the nerve. This explains the variation of cerebral volume with the surface of the body when there is an equal density of innervation, and with the density of innervation when the surface is equal. Now the density of the cutaneous surfaces in the case of man varies very considerably with the region. According to the data of Van Gehuchten, out of about 654,000 fibres of sensibility on each side of the body (the posterior columns of the spinal marrow), of which about 500,000 are concerned with cutaneous sensibility, the division is such that on the average such fibre innervates 1,908 sq. mm. at the head, 1,920 sq. mm. at the upper limb, 2,945 sq.mm. at the lower limb, 3,915 sq. mm. at the trunk. And these values are averages, where the cerebral matter for the finger and the shoulder combine very unequally—to give the common number of the upper limb.

[2] In a case of pure cortical hemianæsthesia through trauma (a fragment of shell) where the skull had been driven in to the level of the upper region of the ascending parietal, I found that the disturbances extended throughout the body except the mucous membrane and the genital organs. The receptive elements of those parts—which would furnish thalamic impressions especially—being situated on the inter-hemispherical surface, would presumably be less vulnerable. At the level of the median lines of separation of the two halves of the body we find lesser disturbances encroaching a little on the opposite side. On the median side there is evidently a confusion of the two lateral innervations, each corresponding to a decussation of the hemisphere.

bility, can alone reveal incomplete and diffuse disturbances, undiscoverable in the region of the upper part of the limbs, whose sensibility remains more crude.

Without providing injuries as limited as those that can be produced by the scalpel, wounds due to projectiles have, much more often than the habitual accidents of human pathology, caused pure and localized sensory disturbances, and have thus confirmed previous views of the sensory topography of the cortex.

2. *Topographic Relations of the Various Forms of Cutaneous and Deep Sensibility*

Psycho-physiological analysis has led us to distinguish the independent forms of cutaneous sensibility and deep sensibility. We shall retain the following: touch, properly speaking (cutaneous to a light pressure), and deep touch (pressures exercising their effect on the sub-cutaneous regions, the muscles, etc.); thermal sensibility for cold and heat, both cutaneous; the so-called pain-sensibility with distinct forms for pricking, burning and bruising (cutaneous and deep); sensibility through bone revealed by vibratory stimuli; and finally the sensibility known as kinæsthetic, or arthro-muscular (movements and resistances).

The sense of position and tactile discrimination, which imply complex reactions, are often also treated as forms of elementary sensibility.

How do the various forms of sensibility, whose independence is shown in the conduction paths of the medullary bundles and in the relay stations, behave from the point of view of the topography of cortical representation.

In this respect a clinical view of the character of anæsthesias of cortical origin would seem to imply a very incomplete representation.

Verger, in 1909, on the evidence of forty cases, twenty

of which were based upon anatomical examination, stated that after lesions of the cerebral hemispheres, pain and the thermal sensations were little affected, that the tactile sense was affected 'qualitatively' in particular, chiefly from the point of view of localization, that stereognosis—called 'active touch'—was constantly diminished or destroyed, as well as the sense of position ("the idea of position of the fingers"); finally that 'akinæsthesia,' that is to say the absence of sensations of movement, was the rule, with persistence of a generalized sensation only.[1]

On the other hand, Dejerine described in 1914 a "sensory cortical syndrome"[2] to which he returned with Mouzon, in January, 1915, in connection with two war cases: this syndrome was characterized by the complete or almost complete integrity of the tactile sense, the integrity of pain and thermal sensations, a perfect or almost perfect preservation of sensation through bone, contrasting with a marked deterioration of the sense of tactile discrimination and of the sense of position, and a constant astereognosis (or loss of the tactile appreciation of form).

These concordant clinical data suggest a cortical representation almost entirely limited to kinæsthetic sensibility.

But the war cases, which multiplied cortical anæsthesias, showed that the "sensory cortical syndrome" had by no means an absolute value. And, towards the end of 1915, Dejerine and Mouzon described a "new type of sensory cortical syndrome" almost the opposite of the first.[3]

Having myself studied in some detail several cases

[1] Verger, "Sur les troubles de la sensibilité générale consécutifs aux lésions des hémisphères cérébraux chez l'homme," *Archives Générales de Médecine*, 1900, p. 513 and p. 662.

[2] Dejerine, *Séméiologie des affections du système nerveux*, 1914.

[3] J. Dejerine and J. Mouzon, "Un nouveau type de syndrome sensitif cortical observé dans un cas de monoplégie corticale dissociée," *Revue Neurologique*, 1915, XXII, pp. 1265-1273.

of cortical anæsthesia resulting from war lesions, one of which was a very good example of pure hemianæsthesia, I prepared a summary of typical French observations during the war, though they were unfortunately as a rule inadequate as regards analysis of the disturbances. I also endeavoured to estimate the frequency and intensity of the injury to the forms of sensibility and to the elementary modes of perception, often confounded with the sensations themselves.[1]

Attributing to each sensation a coefficient running from 1 (considered normal) to 5 (complete disappearance), the mean coefficients of the observations collected give:

Sensation:	Superficial Touch	3·60
	Deep Pressure	3·54
	Heat and Cold	3·21
	Pain	3·35
	Vibration through Bone	3·47
	Appreciation of Weight	3·75
Perception:	Tactile Discrimination	3·80
	Tactile Localization	3·38
	Position	4·00
	Stereognosis	4·13

Though these statistics are only approximate and are generally based on rather rough clinical examinations, the disturbances seem, on an average, to affect all forms of elementary sensibility and perception; but the sense of position is most often and most completely affected; it is only exceptionally normal.

Thermal sensibility and sensibility to pain are the most frequently unaffected or relatively unaffected, but

[1] *Cf.* H. Piéron, "La question des localisations sensitives de l'écorce et le syndrome sensitif cortical," *Revue de Médecine*, 1919, pp. 129-157. French publications of similar observations since this date, and such foreign publications as I am acquainted with, only confirm the results of my statistical statement. (*Cf.* Rose, *Rev. Neur.*, 1921, p. 191; Roussy, d'Œlsnitz and Cornil, *Rev. Neur.*, 1919, p. 311; De Sanctis, *Rivista Ospedaliera*, Sept. 18, 1919; Brunschweiler, *Etabl. sanitaire de Lucerne*, 1919, p. 243, etc.)

contrary to Landberg's[1] statement, this need not always be true; and besides, we should note that sensibility to pain is generally explored only for prick, which is significant.

More careful examinations have been made, however, by Head and Holmes in four cases of operations on tumours in the post-Rolandic region.[2]

According to their results, in cortical anæsthesia touch is not affected: there is only great variability of sensation, with a considerable elevation of the threshold under the influence of fatigue through repetition of the tests. Sensibility to pain is not in the least affected, and the threshold for prick is not modified. Thermal sensibility to hot and cold is only a little less delicate (enlargement of the neutral area), but not in a constant way. The appreciation of posture and of movement is frequently disturbed, especially at the extremities. Localization is often less exact, and delicacy of discrimination is always parallel to it. Appreciation of weight generally has a wide margin of error. Perception of size and form is only abolished when the sense of posture and tactile sensibility are affected at the same time. Rough and smooth continue to be well recognized, but not fine texture. Finally, the appreciation of vibrations may be diminished, but not abolished.

These conclusions of Head and Holmes were adopted by Monier-Vinard in his interesting report on anæsthesias in cerebral hemiplegia at the congress of French alienists and neurologists at Puy in 1913.[3]

From the detailed examination of the results of Head and Holmes—which give us no information at all concerning the elementary sensations such as deep pressure and pain—we may infer, as a whole, that there was an

[1] "Uber die Sensibilitätstörungen bei cerebralen Hemiplegie," *Deutsche Zeitschr. für Nervenheilkunde*, 1906, XXX, pp. 149-166.

[2] Head and G. Holmes, "Sensory disturbances from cerebral lesions," *Brain*, 1912, XXXIV, pp. 102-254.

[3] *Cf. Revue Neurologique*, 1913, XXVI, pp. 209-220.

unequal but very general injury of the various forms of sensibility; and these authors explain the nature of this injury by an attractive hypothesis to which we shall return.

Prickly pain alone seems to remain, and there is apparently a predominance of the disturbance in the appreciation of posture and of weight, surface and vibratory sensibility being less affected, as in the syndrome of Verger-Déjerine; with this difference, however, that according to Head and Holmes perception (discrimination, localization, and stereognosis) is not invariably disturbed.

Since that time, as a result of a very careful experimental study of parietal war lesions, Head has been led to a somewhat different view, and now admits only a loss of perceptive functions in cortical lesions. He distinguishes three special functions; spatial appreciation, graduation of intensity, and recognition of the nature of the excitation (shape, size, weight and texture).

We shall return to this view, which requires certain reservations.

In fact, numerous war observations have shown that the sensation of pricking itself is fairly often affected by cortical lesions, and that sometimes (second cortical syndrome), superficial sensibility, particularly thermal sensibility, is almost exclusively diminished or abolished. In a case where the cranial parietal bone was broken in, Gerstmann records pain-heat anæsthesia, limited to the ulnar region of the hand, without disturbance of stereognosis and kinæsthesia in the finger-tips.[1]

In an experiment on a very limited lesion produced by a surgical operation (Harvey Cushing), there was thermal hypo-algesia and hypo-æsthesia, and as a consequence an exclusive disturbance of superficial pain-

[1] L. Gerstmann, "Ein Fall von dissoziierter Sensibilitätstörung spinosegmentalen Charakters infolge Hirnverletzung nach Schädelschuss," *Mitteil. der Gesellsch. für inn. Med. in Wien*, 1915, XIV, 13.

heat sensibility on half the hand, with loss of kinæsthesia, however, but on the little finger only. This observation is of great importance, for it establishes the close inter-relation of the connecting neurones of the various forms of sensibility in the representation of the established somatic regions. The frequent disturbance of kinæsthesia in cases of parietal injury, behind the ascending parietal gyrus, also supports the idea of a distinct topographical localization of deep sensibility, which is maintained by pupils of Pierre Marie, such as Chatelin, and to a certain degree, by Mme. Athanassio-Bénisty.[1]

But the fact that, in cerebral hemiplegias, deep sensibility,[2] kinæsthesia, is most commonly injured, certainly indicates a greater vulnerability in this form, which has often been localized in the frontal region, at least in the pre-Rolandic convolution, because its disturbance accompanied injuries not involving the ascending parietal convolution.

It need, then, cause no surprise that in parietal traumata we find, as a distance effect, a slight injury in the postcentral area, producing a disturbance of kinæsthesia. Besides, parietal lesions seem to injure the association path coming from the sensori-motor area and the co-ordinating receptive centres, so that the

[1] *Cf.* Chatelin, *op. cit.*, *Les blessures du cerveau*, 2nd. edit., p. 89 [English translation, *Wounds of the Skull and Brain*, 1918, p. 94]. Mme. Athanassio-Bénisty attributes a somewhat ill-defined rôle of general sensibility, for the whole body, to the parietal lobe, the post-Rolandic convolution serving for the representation of the limbs (for all forms of sensibility): the disturbance would specially concern localization, discrimination, stereognosis and orientation in space. On the whole it would be a matter principally of perceptive disturbances, without topographical representation of the body. There is no evidence for projective representation on the parietal lobe.

[2] Bone sensibility is revealed by vibratory excitation, which can bring into play all the nerve-endings, but excites especially those of the periostium because of the reverberation of the solid support, and it is remarkable how, with cortical dissociation, it follows superficial tactile sensibility, as I have constantly noted, and as H. Krueger has also remarked. ("Ueber Sensibilitätstörungen nach Verletzungen der Grosshirnsrinde," *Zeitschr. Für die ges. Neur. und. Psych.*, 1916, XXXIII).

activity of certain centres is more or less seriously disturbed. The frequent confusion of elementary sensory excitation and complex perceptive judgment, implied, for example, in the idea of a 'sense of position,' leads us to consider defects in the associative functioning of the parietal area,[1] the area of sensory thought, as disturbances of the receptive station.

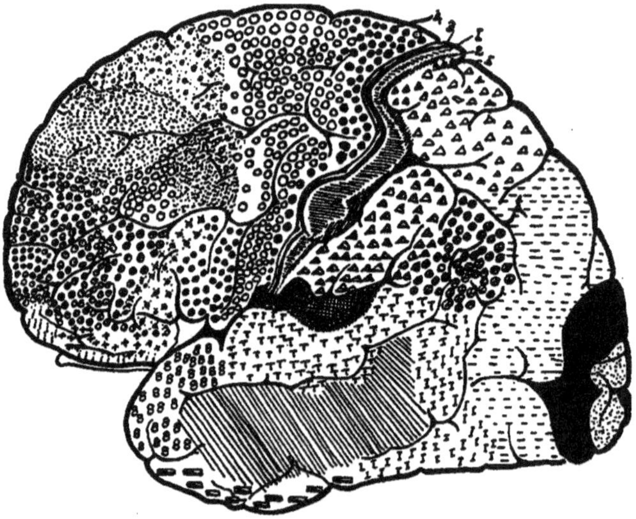

FIG. 8. The architectonic areas of Brodmann (external surface of the left hemisphere).

At 4 we have the area of the motor cortex with the Betz cells; at 1 the sensory area of the post-Rolandic convolution.

It remains to inquire why the different forms of sensibility may be dissociated in this manner in cortical

[1] In one case Minkowski observed disturbances of sensibility in the monkey through extirpation of the parietal area, the ascending parietal being left ntact, but he also obtained it, at first, after the extirpation of the pre-Rolandic, the repair occurring afterwards; but, in this instance, the animal died too soon for repair to be possible. And the ablation of the post-central alone involved permanent disturbance in *all* forms of sensibility aggravated by the simultaneous ablation of the connected parietal area, particularly as regards the localization of the excitations. It is obvious that the interruption of the association path is not unimportant, especially if it is in direct connection with the sub-cortical receptive stations.

lesions ; for in general this dissociation reveals a peculiar vulnerability of the kinæsthesia.[1]

It is possible to suppose that the variation in vulnerability is due to differences in the situation of the connecting neurones connected with the different forms of sensibility. But though we know that the whole ascending parietal convolution corresponds to

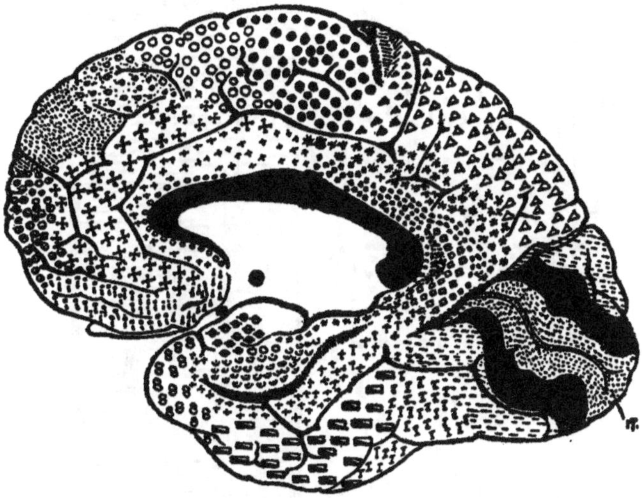

FIG. 9. The architectonic areas of the internal surface. At 17 is indicated the 'area striata' or visual cortex, round the calcarine fissure.

a cortical structure which is not found elsewhere and, in particular, is very different from that which characterizes the motor area of the ascending frontal, and though we also know that it represents a highly individualized structural area, we are not yet in a position to make

[1] An important study by Pierre Marie and Bouttier ("Étude clinique sur les modalités des dissociations de la sensibilité dans les lésions encéphaliques," *Revue neurologique*, XXIX, 1922, pp. 1-22 and pp. 144-160) establishes the fact that all varieties of sensory dissociation can be observed in cortical and sub-cortical lesions, but with a general predominance of injury to deep sensibility, confirming my own analysis, as they are kind enough to remark. They wonder what the mechanism of these dissociations may be, but without offering any definite theory, they reject the explanation in terms of unequal vulnerability.

precise differentiations or localizations as to depth. Experiments on the monkey, when the methods of stimulation or of ablation have been perfected, will doubtless achieve this.

At present we have only hypotheses based on an

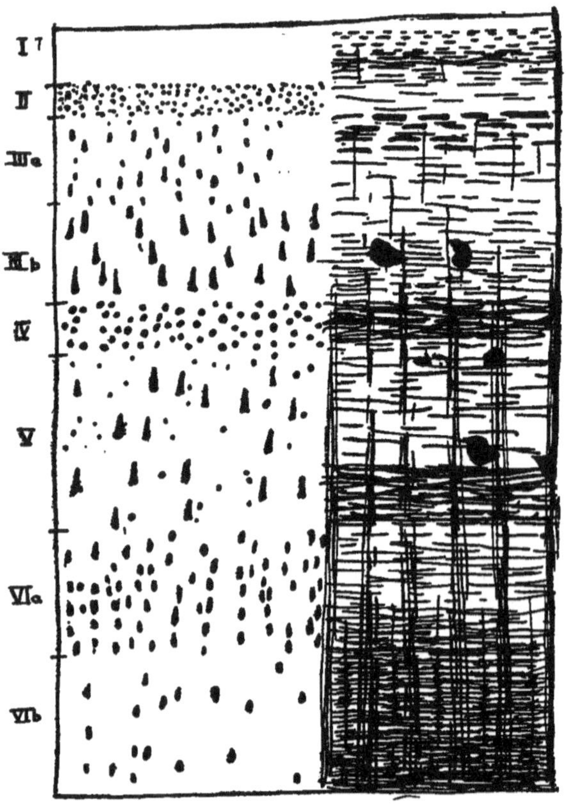

FIG. 10. General diagram of cell strata (cellular-architectonic layers of Brodmann) and the plexuses of fibres (myelo-architectonic of Vogt).

The main layers are: I. the zonal layer, without cells; II. the external granual layer with small cells; III. the pyramidal layer (subdivided into the external region with small cells and the internal region with large cells); IV. the internal granular layer; V. the ganglionic layer with very large pyramidal cells; VI. the multiform layer with polymorph cells.

interpretation of anatomical structures. Ramon y Cajal would place the receptive apparatus for pain, touch and temperature in the layer of the medium-sized pyramidal cells, whence sensations would pass by special tracts into other areas, where they are organized as memories.[1]

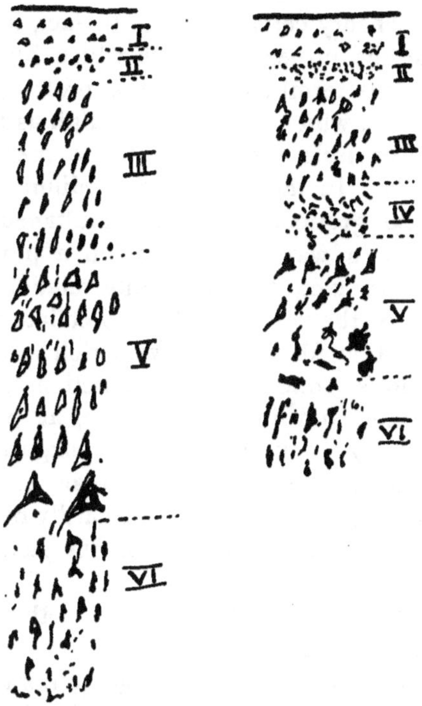

FIG. 11. Diagram of the architectonic of the motor cortex (left) and the sensory cortex (right), after Brodmann.

In the motor cortex, we note the giant Betz cells at the base of layer V, and the absence of layer IV; in the sensory cortex, the layer of the great pyramidal cells is less developed, but layer IV takes an important place.

The psychological theory is questionable, and the localization cannot in any case be admitted, since these receptions would occur in the ascending frontal convolution, which has an exclusively motor function.

[1] S. Ramon y Cajal, *Studien über die Hirnrinde*, 1900.

Rouvière, in an interesting essay on the cerebral cortex,[1] calls attention to the importance of the granular layer, which is absent only in the motor area, and is very well developed in the sensory area, intersecting the layer of large pyramidal cells: these granules, according to him, collect sensations and transmit them to the sensory cells proper. In fact, it is in the granules that the projection fibres which bring in the sensory impulses terminate, and the prolongations of these small cells, which often rise as high as the superficial layers, encircle the body of the medium-sized pyramidal cells. In the small and medium pyramidal cells would be grouped elements simultaneously perceived, in such a way as to occasion a judgment of recognition. In fact, the close interrelation between prolongations of the various cells, and collaterals of the terminal projection fibres, allow very rich associations. But the author's conceptions of function are singularly inadequate, and it is impossible, at present, to rely upon them as a basis for an investigation of the rôle attributed to the different cellular elements in connection with operations which can hardly be regarded as confined to the layers of cells in one small area of the cortex.[2]

We would only note in this connection the considerable area occupied by the third layer of the cortex, containing small, medium and large pyramidal cells, above the fourth or granular layer, which is also very

[1] H. Rouvière, "Essai sur le fonctionnement de l'écorce cérébrale," *Bull. et Mém. de la Soc. d'Anthropologie*, 1919, VIII, pp. 40-66.

[2] In a general way, the middle layers seem to be the seat of connecting neurones (incito-associative sensory reception, for example), the superficial layers seem to be involved in the intellectual associative functions, and finally the deep layers, the first to appear in ontogenetic development, where the projection fibres enter the cortex, seem to serve for the production of the fundamental cortical reactions, and, in particular, of the cortical reflexes (*cf.* J. Shaw Bolton, "A Contribution to the Localization of Cerebral Function, based on the Clinico-pathological Study of Mental Disease," *Brain*, XXXIII, pp. 26-148; "Amentia and Dementia, a Clinico-pathological Study," *Journal of Mental Science*, 1906-07, LII, pp. 1, 221, 427, 711, LIII, p. 84).

highly developed. This suggests the possibility of specialized strata for the connecting neurones influenced by different receptive paths, so that the symptoms may vary according to the region most affected by any lesion. But it is also quite possible that the variation in vulnerability is related to the nature of the connecting neurones, to their own metabolism, rather than to their different situation in the depths of the cortex, if indeed these various groups of neurones are not juxtaposed in minute islets, rather than superposed.

In any case, the reception of all forms of sensibility undoubtedly occurs at a level of the cortex which corresponds to a definite area of the body, and there are no groupings for different forms which can be macroscopically isolated, since their unequal susceptibility occasions variable dissociations after cortical lesions.

3. *Perceptive Functions and Receptive Co-ordination*

Perception is more affected than sensation by cortical lesions of the sensory area. But is it legitimate to make a radical distinction between sensation and perception? In reality, any impression whatever implies a perception, of varying precision but undeniable. If I am touched on the right arm and I feel something, I can at least indicate the approximate region of the body involved, if not the exact place of the contact. I do not confuse the foot with the head, and I am sure that it is a matter of a contact, not of an odour or a light, even without being able to state the exact nature of this contact. As soon as a sensation is definitely felt, an excitation received really is occasioning an associative reaction, which includes the evocation of representations and verbal symbols, the taking of attitudes, and, if necessary, motor reactions. But when we speak of perceptive function we are referring to high degrees of this function of elementary thought, which have become delicate and exact, as distinguished from the crude manifestations which are never absent if there is really a definite sensation.

Now, just as finely graduated movements are always rendered impossible by injuries of the incito-motor region of the cortex, so with lesions of the incito-associative area it is the precise and finely differentiated evocations which are the first to be affected and the last to re-establish themselves, provided these lesions, while causing more or less permanent functional disturbances, have not involved definite destructions.

If a point on the wrist of the right hand is touched, and then another very near it, and if the connecting neurones excited in the cortical area each bring into action a definite associative circuit and accurately call forth the appropriate representations and reactions, each of the points will be perceived as distinct from the other, and will be localized with fair success by a gesture or a description in visual terms.

In order that these highly discriminative associations may be possible, there must be in the inter-connection of the neurones a sort of exact syntonization between the neurones of the circuit, in conformity with conclusions which certainly seem to be implied by the latest view of elementary nervous functioning, in consequence of the researches of Lapicque and his pupils.[1]

But when even a slight disturbance occurs in the functioning of a neurone, there is an alteration in its own appropriate coefficient of emission of impulses, and this alteration, correlated no doubt with a modification of metabolism, will show itself in its relations with the other groups of neurones: it will no longer be selected, as it was before; and it will act in an unqualified way with a more intense operation on the various groups of neurones; a precise redirection of

[1] See later, in Chapter V, an outline of the principal data on the functional operation of the neurones in the selective reactions.

its associative impulse will no longer be possible. Thereafter, localization will become uncertain and discrimination will require stimuli which are so far removed that the corresponding connecting neurones can no longer so easily intermingle their respective ill-directed evocations.

It is clear, then, for a given category of sensations, that so long as what we call crude sensibility is not noticeably diminished and the usual intensities of excitation are still capable of provoking a response, perceptive power may be affected and the selectivity of the response may lose its precision;[1] differential sensibility, which though quantitative is more especially qualitative, and which is the basis of cerebral functioning and really conditions all mental processes, is first and most seriously affected.

But in the dissociations we have mentioned, a given mode of sensibility may sometimes remain sufficiently unaffected for even its perceptive functioning to be satisfactory—for example, discrimination between two cutaneous contacts or two hot or cold stimulations, etc. On the other hand, analogous perceptions result from different forms of sensibility: discrimination between two superficial contacts may be difficult and unqualified, while that between two painful prick stimuli remains delicate; localization of a light contact may be uncertain while localization of a deep pressure is still fairly accurate.

An examination of the perceptive functions requires experimental precautions rarely observed with sufficient care in clinical experiments.

Finally, there are perceptions which require the

[1] In cortical injuries, at least in those which do not involve very extensive or very complete destructions, there may be a re-education of perception, which Graham Brown has described, especially with regard to localization, in war cases. (*Cf.* T. Graham Brown and R. M. Stewart, "On Disturbances of the Localization and Discrimination of Sensations in Cases of Cerebral Lesions, and on the Possibility of Recovery of these Functions after a Process of Training," *Brain*, 1916, XXXIX, pp. 348-454).

participation of at least two forms of sensibility; namely, perceptions of shape, in active exploration with the fingers. I recognize a cylinder which I feel in my hand by the even pressure on the pulp of my fingers when I roll it, while my kinæsthetic sense gives me information concerning the movements that I make in causing it to roll. This occurs when I roll it in one direction, but when I try to make it roll in a perpendicular direction I fail, and am aware of it: I find a single contact, I draw it towards me with a sliding movement, then suddenly a flexion of the finger is necessary in order to preserve the contact, and I find a new homogeneous surface, which I explore. When the impressions appear symmetrically the same at both extremities, all this complex whole arouses the representation of the cylinder.

But if my kinæsthetic impressions become very crude or are almost abolished, my awkward exploration, though my tactile sensations retain their delicacy, will not allow a satisfactory identification; I may sometimes guess correctly, but I shall make errors. If my tactile sensibility alone is affected, I can still, even with crude impressions, obtain very exact ideas of form, so long as my kinæsthetic sense remains delicate, especially if sensations of deep pressure supplement the superficial contact. But if I am completely deprived of tactile sensations and sensations of pressure, I shall no longer perceive forms. Also stereognosis, the perception of form, can frequently be diminished or abolished in cortical lesions which sometimes—indeed, usually—involve the loss of kinæsthesia, and sometimes the loss of tactile sensibility, when the two forms of sensibility are not simultaneously affected. But, in certain cases, it has been noticed that stereognosis alone has been abolished, and its abolition has been connected with certain parietal lesions. Is there then a stereognostic centre, analogous to the centres of elementary sensibility, as certain authors think—Senise for example, who, moreover, would place it in the ascending parietal convolution?[1] It is certainly true that stereognosis is often less exact in parietal injuries, without lesions of the post-Rolandic receptive convolution, and is generally accompanied by very little delicacy of discrimination and tactile localization.

This might be simply a distance effect on the receptive area, a slight injury reappearing in the most delicate and susceptible perceptive functioning. On the other hand, it is certain that the parietal region is that of the association paths emanating from the receptive station; it is there that the association circuits include the greatest number of relay neurones and switches. A cortical lesion in this region must therefore necessarily provoke in these association circuits a disturbance of 'tactile thought,' and hence of spatial representation of the skin and the power of recognizing shapes. This does not mean that we may locate there the 'centres' of perception as distinct from the centres of sensibility. Perception is a complex dynamic act which is not readily located; but the dynamism has a support, and an injury to the chief nerve tracts in a given region will inevitably produce functional disturbances.

But is there nothing further?

A key is put into my hand; I say: "It is a key." I have not even examined its shape, I recognize it immediately. And, if I analyse my impressions, I only do so afterwards. This is a 'gnosis,' the recognition of a common object, as distinct from 'stereognosis,' the perception of shape, though they are commonly confused. And, in fact, in certain cases the shape is correctly perceived and described, while the object is not recognized nor can its name be recalled, and it is even impossible to indicate, by gesture or by appropriate use, that its practical employment and purpose are known. But at other times, with very defective perception of

[1] *Annali di Nevrologia*, 1918, XXXIV, pp. 113-144.

shapes, common objects are indicated, successfully guessed [1] and correctly handled.

Here we are far from the sensory area, and are entering the intellectual area: the selective associative reaction, aroused—sometimes erroneously—by various sensory signs (the coldness of the metal playing an important part, for example, in the perception of the key) and characteristic of the concrete idea of the object, is easier and quicker than the perception of its shape constructed on a complex synthesis of immediate impressions.

For these common objects immediately recognized and automatically named—though confusion is often easy—we must admit the existence of a co-ordinating station which is quite ready, under the influence of certain definite stimuli, to put into operation the usual reactions, a word, an action or a posture. An injury at the level of this co-ordinating station would thus involve a pure 'agnosia' and 'an agnosic apraxia,' the incapacity to make the movements required for the handling of an object (pen-holder, scissors, etc.), but only because the object is not recognized; and all this occurs without sensory disturbances, with correct perception if the incito-associative area is not damaged, and without motor or general intellectual disturbances.[2] With regard to the exact location of this gnosic co-ordination centre (which would be a true centre of perception or at least of symbolic perception), the data relative to pure agnosias, unfortunately very rare, suggest that it is situated in the parietal region of one hemisphere only, usually the left. Gnosic disorders frequently accompany

[1] In his description of 'tactile blindness,' Niessl von Mayendorf rightly distinguishes loss of perception, accompanying anterior cortical lesions, from loss of the power of identification and of associative evocation which characterizes more posterior lesions ("Tastblindheit," *Zeitschrift für die gesamte Neurologie*, 1919, L, p. 82).

[2] There are in fact demential agnosias which constitute only one of the symptoms of intellectual injury or general inadequacy of associative functioning.

general disturbances of symbolic thought of which general aphasia is the most obvious manifestation, and also certain disturbances of verbal symbolic co-ordination upon which we shall have more to say when we come to discuss the cerebral function of language.

4. *Rôle and Significance of Cortical Reception in the Sensori-motor Cycle*

When a sensory excitation reaches the cortex, it has already entered into connection with a series of superposed centres of reflex association and has called forth groups of appropriate local or general reactions, connected with the cycle of vegetative life or even on that of integrative action.

If I step into cold water, I feel well-defined thermal sensations; but before calling forth the associative reactions and reflexes of recognition, the cutaneous excitation has aroused at the level of the spinal cord and the bulb vaso-motor and thermogenic reactions; the blood-vessels of the lower limb have undergone a relatively intense constriction, the production of heat liberated in the organism by the liver and the muscles has been increased and a bristling of the hairs has produced 'goose-flesh.' All these manifestations will persist even when I do not perceive the cold, and even though the intellectual reaction, the registering of the experience for the future, be lacking. In the absence of any transmission to the cortical centres of excitation, if the foot is dipped into boiling water, a retractive movement will occur in the lower limb, and if it is kept there, movements of the other limb, of motor agitation, will succeed.

Let us note the behaviour of Dusser de Barenne's cats, with the cortex removed but the sub-cortical centres and thalamus still intact: they withdraw their paws from cold or hot water, but only when the water is very cold or very hot, and after a considerable time; they react when their hair is touched, avoiding an obstacle, after several days of adaptation, directly their whiskers brush it; they walk correctly, without ataxia, move their ears in response to a whistle, and protect themselves when pinched, but awkwardly, with faulty localization.

Thus—with a minimum of precision in the reaction, which remains momentary and ceases with the stimulus instead of influencing the later behaviour of the animal—the decerebrate cat presents responses which are not only vegetative but also integrative, not only partial but also general.

Whether this implies psychical activity need not be discussed, if by 'psychical' we understand a conscious reverberation—for the problem is insoluble. We can, however, affirm that it does not involve association, with that awakening of imagery, that complex elaboration of reactions, which may be regarded as characteristic of psychical life.

We may assume, therefore, that these sub-cortical responses remain just as foreign to psychical life, to thought, as the thermogenic and vaso-motor reactions, and that, furthermore, when cortical functioning is ensured, an inhibition of these responses allows only the precise and elaborated reactions of the higher area to persist.

But another question arises, as a result of the classic experiments of Head. Are there not among the sensory excitations that arouse unqualified sub-cortical responses, some which, instead of ending in the receptive centres of the cortex, cease at the lower level, and yet are the object of knowledge? Could the knowledge of these stimuli occur at this sub-cortical level? This Head seems to assume; but knowledge at once implies a certain associative reaction, a direct involvement of the circuits of the higher area. Hence it seems certain that the thalamus, where some receptive impulses terminate, must contain associatively incited neurones, less numerous and less susceptible to fine shades of evocation, but entering into relation with the whole intellectual area of the cortex.

Just as there are direct relations between the associative area and the incito-motor nuclei of the intermediate levels, without passing through the incito-motor station of the cortex, which are revealed by persistence of voluntary motor behaviour after the destruction of this last station, so we may assume that there are direct relations between the sub-cortical receptive nuclei and the associative area, and not passing through the cortical receptive area.

And, in fact, the destruction of the receptive station of one hemisphere fails to suppress completely either the immediate reactivity, or even the knowledge of the cutaneous or deep sensory excitations, as shown in verbal reaction or adaptive behaviour.

Perhaps even the real loss of sensibility might be less if there were not certain possible distance reverberations from the terminal exhaustion, reaching to the nearest of the lower levels.

Minkowski's monkeys with the ascending parietal convolution removed, and sometimes the rest of the parietal lobe as well, showed a quantitative but more especially a qualitative diminution of the tactile sense, of sensibility to cold and heat; the thresholds were higher, the perceptions cruder, and the localization incorrect; kinæsthetic sensibility was disturbed, but sensibility to pain was hardly affected, and in particular the localization of the painful excitations remained fairly exact. In the case of man, in the most complete cortical hemianæsthesia, strong pressure is still felt, there is awareness of intense cold and excessive heat, while sensibility to pain—though it may be diminished or retarded, often to a remarkable extent—is never abolished, especially for stimuli other than pricking (pinching or burning).

We must then assume a sensory knowledge which does not imply that the connecting agents of the cortical receptive area enter the circuits of the associative area. A series of association paths linking the thalamus with different levels of the cortex, and others, inversely, connecting the cortex to the thalamus, make this direct relation anatomically possible, in addition to the system of projection fibres which conducts sensory impulses to the cortex, where they are themselves transmitted from neurone to neurone at the different levels where reflex co-ordination takes place.

How then does Head conceive of the division between thalamic and cortical reception in the different forms of sensibility?

Without entering into the details of the facts which he has recorded with such force and originality, let us briefly indicate the main lines of the system which he has gradually elaborated, though we shall not be able to accept it in its entirety.

The facts have emerged from an experimental analysis —conceived on purely physiological lines—of sensory disturbances due to injuries of peripheral nerves, spinal conduction tracts, bulbar tracts and sub-cortical centres, and of the cortex itself.[1]

Injury of a peripheral nerve reveals curious dissociations of sensibility which a bold experiment—since repeated by various physiologists—enabled Head to observe very closely. A sensory nerve of his forearm was divided (the external cutaneous nerve, and the superficial branch of the radial), and during the experiments conducted by his collaborator, the late W. H. R. Rivers, a well-known psycho-physiologist, he noted the initial state of sensibility in the area rendered an-

[1] *Cf.* W. H. Rivers and Henry Head, "A Human Experiment in Nerve Division," *Brain*, XXXI, 3, 1908, pp. 323-450.—Head and Sherren, "The Consequences of Injury to the Peripheral Nerves in Man," *Brain*, XXVIII, 2, 1905, pp. 116-338.—Head, Rivers and Sherren, "The Afferent Nervous System from a New Aspect," *Brain*, XXVIII, 1, 1905, pp. 99-115.—Head and Thompson, "The Grouping of Afferent Impulses within the Spinal Cord," *Brain*, XXIX, 4, 1907, pp. 537-741.—Head and Holmes, "Sensory Disturbances from Cerebral Lesions," *Brain*, XXXIV, 2-3, 1911, pp. 102-254.

æsthetic and its neighbourhood, and then the stages of its return during the nerve regeneration. He distinguished, besides the deep sensibility to touch that persisted despite superficial anæsthesia, two types of cutaneous sensibility, 'protopathic' and 'epicritic.'

Thus heat and cold can be felt by either system. Protopathic sensation—the first to reappear during recovery—requires a very great difference in temperature between the stimulus and the skin ; the sensation evoked is very painful and diffuse, and badly localized ; there is no delicate differentiation of intensity ; especially when epicritic sensibility has not yet reappeared, its painful and even intolerable character provokes vigorous reactions.

Sensations of heat and cold subserved by the epicritic system are evoked by slight differences in temperature. The sensations are indifferent, well localized and delicately graduated.

Cutaneous excitation with the point of a needle, when protopathic sensibility alone has reappeared, produces also a vague and diffuse impression, very painful and badly localized ; on the other hand, after a return of epicritic sensibility, the contact is accurately localized, discrimination between the contacts of two neighbouring points is delicate and the painful impression is, to some extent, inhibited.

The conductors of the two varieties of sensibility are distinct in the main nerve-stem, the protopathic conductors behaving in a different way, during recovery, from the epicritic conductors.

In the spinal cord, a regrouping of the sensory tracts takes place ; the conductors of the thermal sensations, epicritic and protopathic, are reunited and travel together, and in thermal anæsthesia for cold or heat alone, or for both heat and cold, we no longer find the feature which we observe in lesions of the nerves.

On the other hand new features appear ; epicritic sensibility travels by different paths from discriminatory sensibility (in the appreciation of two points) and from stereognosis, with which the paths of deep kinæsthetic sensibility are related.

In the brain-stem and the thalamus the features of peripheral protopathic and epicritic sensations reappear, and new characters are found in epicritic tactile sensibility; the appreciation of roughness and localization may be separately affected.

The termination of the various sensibilities confirms the dissociation. Epicritic sensibility to hot and cold, which is not dissociable, epicritic touch, discriminatory and stereognostic sensibility, localization, and kinæsthetic sensibility ascend as far as the cortex. Protopathic sensibility to hot and cold, cutaneous pain, deep pain, the tactile appreciation of roughness, and the appreciation of vibration through bone, pass no further than the thalamus. We can group these data diagrammatically—

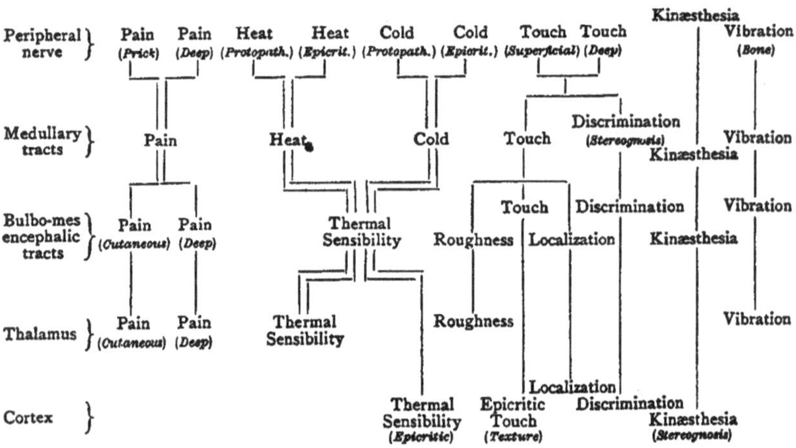

But this interesting arrangement cannot be accepted in all its details. On the one hand it is constructed as though we were dealing with elementary sensations, and introduces complex perceptive functions which would never be supposed to have medullary or bulbo-mesencephalic conductors: discrimination, or stereognosis, localization, and the idea of roughness or texture of bodies. Such distinctions are based on the interpretation of certain disturbances (particularly in Brown-Séquard syndromes[1]) which by no means bear out the conclusions that Head has drawn from them.

On the other hand, numerous analyses of nervous lesions during the war and repeated experiments in the autosection of sensory branches prevent our admitting Head's protopathic sensibility in the exact form he has given it.[2]

[1] Brown-Séquard's syndrome is due to a hemisection of the spinal cord, all the conductors of the right or of the left side being interrupted. As the conductors of the various sensibilities pass into the opposite half of the spinal cord at different levels, such a section interrupts the homolateral tracts not yet crossed and the heterolateral tracts after crossing. Both halves of the body are then affected, but for different sensibilities. Tactile impressions however, are divided into two bundles, one of which crosses as soon as it enters the spinal cord while the other ascends on the same side; there is never a complete abolition of touch; the inequality of the bundles involves, however, an almost complete abolition of one side and a slight injury to the other side which is enough to disturb discrimination and which, co-existing with the kinæsthetic injury, abolishes stereognosis. There can be no question of finding special conductors of discrimination, for this occurs with prickly pain, impressions of hot and cold or deep pressure, as well as with tactile stimuli (*Cf.* H. Piéron, "De la discrimination spatiale des sensations thermiques. Son importance pour la théorie générale de la discrimination cutanée," *C. R. Soc. Biologie,* 1919, LXXXII, pp. 61-65.—C. Spearman, "Analysis of Localization illustrated by a Brown-Séquard Case," *British Journal of Psychology,* 1905, I, 3, pp. 284-314).

[2] *Cf.* Harvey Carr, "Head's Theory of Cutaneous Sensibility," *Psychological Review,* 1916, XXIII, 4, pp. 262-278 (Discussion).—M. von Frey "Beobachtungen an Hautflächen mit geschädigter Innervation," *Zeitschr. für Biol.* 1914, LXIII, pp. 335-370 (An examination of the cutaneous area with an anomaly of innervation).—F. Hacker, "Ein Beitrag zum Studium der Regeneration von Hautnerven," *Z. f. Biol.,* 1915, LXV, pp. 67-78 (Study of the lesion of a nerve of the forearm by an injection of iodine).—W. Trotter and H. M. Davies, "Experimental Studies in the Innervation of the Skin," *Journal of Physiology,* 1909, XXXVIII, pp. 134-246; "The Peculiarities of Sensibility found in Cutaneous Areas supplied by Regenerating Nerves," *Journal für Psychologie und Neurologie,* 1913, XX, Erg. Heft 2, pp. 102-150 (Important researches with experimental section, in trained subjects of seven different cutaneous nerve branches; all the sensory functions made a parallel reappearance but there were phenomena of intensification and a disturbance of reference).—E. G. Boring, "Cutaneous Sensation after Nerve-division," *Quarterly Journal of experimental Physiology,* 1916, X,

From these results we see that beyond the hyperalgesia which appears in regions deprived of their normal innervation, either at the beginning or at an early stage of regeneration, we can give no evidence of really distinct protopathic sensibility.

To sum up: there is a pain sense which is called forth by extreme heat or cold (Boring), which corresponds to Head's protopathic sensibility and is a sensibility to burning of a specific character; there is also a deep pain sense which is not abolished by section of the cutaneous nerves, and a cutaneous pain sense of prick (not considering a possible cutaneous sensibility to pinching or bruising). Head's observations are doubtless forms of pain sense, or rather of algesic reactivity, affective and very intense, such as is revealed by 'causalgia' in peripheral nerve lesions.[1]

And this vague, diffuse and intolerable pain-reactivity seems to occur in certain thalamic injuries, evidently of an irritative character, in consequence of cerebral lesions. Hemianæsthesia through lesion of the thalamus, interrupting the projection tracts which enter the cortex after this

pp. 1-95 (A study of autosection of the anterior branch of the internal cutaneous nerve of the forearm; introspective distinctions; the preservation of deep impressions; no protopathic dissociation; phenomena of hyperalgesia in regeneration, especially for thermal stimuli).—L. T. Pollock, "Nerve Overlap as related to the Relatively Early Return of Pain Sense following Injury to the Peripheral Nerves," *Journal of Comparative Neurology*, 1920, XXXII, pp. 357-378 (Observations on 500 cases of peripheral nerve lesions. The early return of pain sensibility is connected with a hyperalgesic phenomenon in the region of adjacent nerves).

[1] In causalgia, there is an irritation of sympathetic fibres—in very capricious directions, following the trunks of the nerves, and particularly the arterial coats—causing extreme erethism of the centres of painful reactivity, which very easily reaches a crisis under the influence of sensory action and even under the influence of psychic action. The pain seems like burning (Weir Mitchell's 'thermalgia'), which suggests that this form of pain—combined with Head's protopathic thermal sensibility may be transmitted by the unmyelinated sympathetic fibres (*Cf.* W. Ranson, "Unmyelinated Nerve-fibres as Conductors of Protopathic Sensation," *Brain*, 1915, XXXVIII, 3, pp. 381-389.—Ranson and Billingsley, "The Conduction of Painful Afferent Impulses in the Spinal Nerves," *Am. J. of Physiology* 1916, XL, pp. 571-584.—J. Tinel, "Contribution a l'étude de l'origine sympathique de la causalgie," *Rev. Neu. o'ogique*, 1917, XXIV, (2), pp. 243-255).

last stage, is usually accompanied by frequent painful crises, the pain remains diffuse, indeterminate, and localized very badly or not at all, as in causalgic crises, and in general is of a very distressing character.[1]

These data, even if they somewhat modify Head's general scheme, are in any case in full agreement with the principles on which it is based. The thalamus is a centre of affective reactivity to sensory stimuli, while the cortex is an apparatus for discrimination.[2]

Before determining the particular functions of the thalamic and cortical levels, in the elaboration of responses to stimuli, let us diagrammatize in a revised form the data relative to the principle divisions of general sensibility, which might be classified, in accordance with Sherrington's grouping, as 'proprioceptive,' when they give information specially concerning the modifications undergone by the organism (painful sensations or kinæsthesia), and 'exteroceptive' when they give information especially concerning an exterior agent (touch or temperature).

The thalamus, which in the lower vertebrates deprived of the cortex ensures the general reactions of the organism and the elementary mental functions,[3] possesses an

[1] See, for example, the observations of Faure-Beaulieu and Aymès: "Syndrome thalamique traumatique," *Revue Neurologique*, 1918 (XXV (20) 7-8, pp. 10-14) and of Guillain ("Syndrome thalamique consécutif à une blessure de guerre," *Bull. Soc. Médicale des Hôpitaux*, 1917, XLI, pp. 1110-1114).

[2] These reservations as to the existence of the thalamic sensory centres have been adopted by Pierre Marie and Bouttier, who admit affective reverberation only at the level of the thalamus. "Our clinical researches," they say, "result in conclusions agreeing, on the whole, with those of M. Piéron" (*loc. cit.* p. 144).

[3] C. J. Herrick, who allows that the cortex co-ordinates and integrates sub-cortical circuits, in which the sensory data become impregnated with thalamic affective elements, among the higher mammals, considers that among the lower vertebrates (fishes and bactracians) the thalamus is the organ of the highest associations (adaptation and the rudiments of associative memory) governed by smell and sight, Edinger's neothalamus appearing as a vestibule which establishes communication with the cortex (*Cf.* C. Judson Herrick, "Some Reflections on the Origin and Significance of the Central Cortex," *Journal of Animal Behaviour*, 1913, III, 3, pp. 222-236.—"A Sketch of the Origin of the Cerebral Hemispheres," *J. of Comparative Neurology*, 1921, XXXII, 4, pp. 429-454.) We may also note that in the case of the decerebrate cat (Dusser de Barenne) the existence of the thalamus enables the animal to learn to avoid obstacles, from the data furnished by the whiskers.

affective excitability in relation with the profound biological tendencies of the organism; among the higher mammals, indeed, it seems to preserve this rôle of affective regulation, whose importance in the behaviour of the organism and mental life is so often misunderstood; we shall return to this point.

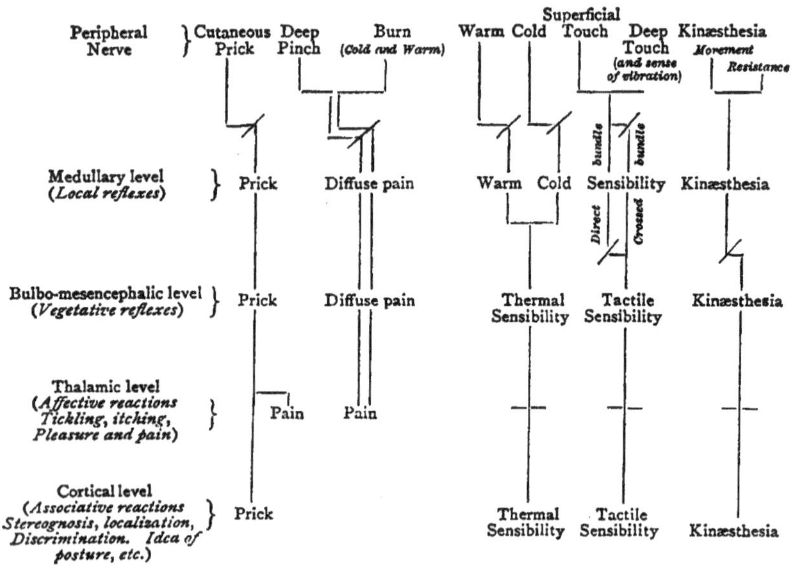

In this diagram, when the line depicting the paths of conduction forms an angle cut by a diagonal line, it indicates that the crossing occurs at this level—the passage from one side of the body to the other; the tactile paths undergo decussation at two different levels.

Normally the sensory excitations perceived by the cortex are accompanied by affective excitations aroused in the sub-cortical centre, and reappearing in their turn in the associative area where their influence must be considerable. In the mental mechanism, this special influence of the sub-cortical reactions would not be negligible, since it is constantly present. And conversely, when normal equilibrium is not disturbed, the associative area exercises a considerable inhibitory influence on affective reactivity at a lower level. We must remember, for example, the rôle that psychical inhibition or reinforcement may play in the reverberation produced by an excitation, in itself very moderate, of the cutaneous receptors of the armpit or the sole of the foot, and known as tickling; both in our intellectual reaction and our symbolic representation we thus confuse the sensory excitation itself with the entire affective and motor complex which it calls forth.

A sensation of 'pain' is also in reality a combination of sensation and affective reaction—a fact which is still often overlooked, in spite of the individuality given to 'sensations of pain' by the analysis of sensory points and medullary conductors.

This individuality proves conclusively that not all the receptors are capable of arousing a painful reaction, and also shows that certain receptors, when stimulated, produce a comparatively intense affective reaction, of modifiable quality, itching or tickling—and perhaps even sexual pleasure also—constituting as a whole the first manifestations of the receptive systems of pain.

These receptive systems only enter into thought as a result of affective reverberation, with the sole exception of pricking, in which the character of discriminatory sensation realized at the level of the cortical area is fairly well isolated from the painful reverberation (when this latter is not too exaggerated, as in the protopathic stage of nerve regeneration, in causalgia, the irritative thalamic syndrome, etc.). In contradistinction to deep pain through pinching and the irradiations of burning, pricking allows localization and discrimination as exact and delicate as that of touch, although the receptive and conductive systems are entirely different and easily dissociable.

In the absence of the cortical receptive station which, thanks to the plurality of cutaneous receptors at the surface of the upper layer of the skin, permits of specific associative reactions producing local qualities, we have only the indirect information furnished by the thalamic reactions to sufficiently strong stimuli, and by the disagreeable or painful impressions experienced in connection with special stimuli: 'exteroceptive' sensibility becomes a sort of cœnæsthesia, and organic impressions ('interoceptive' sensibility) appear in all cases to arrive at the cortex only when translated by the thalamus, with its own affective elaboration.

When a limb is affected by cortical anæsthesia, in the absence of continuous small excitations, it is curious to note how far this limb is forgotten, unknown and carried like a foreign body. It appears to be paralysed,[1] although its movements remain possible and correct, and the paralysis even seems considerably more serious than in cases of hemiplegia without anæsthesia, where the patient, who is awkward with his limb, generally makes an effort to use it and is to a certain extent successful. Except under violent stimulation, which is rare, or where the thalamus recalls to the cortex the existence of the limb, nothing reminds the patient that this limb can still be made use of. This is in strong contrast with cases where the amputated limb is really alive, through the intermediation of the corresponding sensory area which constantly impinges on the associative circuits of kinæsthetic and tactile thought, with its

[1] This is the 'psychic paralysis' of Bruns, often noticed during the war, in pure and complete sensory monoplegias due to a localized lesion of the ascending parietal and already recorded after slight injuries (*Cf.* for example, André Thomas, "Abcès du lobe pariétal," *Revue Neurologique*, 1913, XXI, 10, pp. 637-652).

We may observe that there is no real 'ataxia' in the movements of one limb when cortical kinæsthesia is absent; habitual movements are well executed, and the necessary control of the kinæsthetic impressions is effected at the level of the sub-cortical centres. It is only when this control is lacking that ataxia appears. Head has emphasized this sub-cortical realization of motor co-ordination through kinæsthetic regulation. Cases have been recently reported of ataxia, through injury to the sub-cortical mechanism, coexisting with preservation of the power of movement and of superficial and deep sensibility, in an incomplete cerebral hemiplegia (*Cf.*, Monier-Vinard and Longchampt, "Monoplégie brachiale dissociée avec inco-ordination motrice," *Revue Neurologique*, 1922, XXXVIII, 3, pp. 317-320).

memories of impressions. These latter are often aroused by the irritations which it undergoes, at the level of the scar, since the nervous conductors have remained in connection with the specific receptors.[1]

When cortical anæsthesia accompanies the destruction of the incito-motor area, the limb may remain totally forgotten, as in the case of a monkey reported by Minkowski, where he had made a total ablation of the right centro-parietal region: "If not only the right arm, but also the head of the animal was rendered immoveable," he says, "for three months it still did not make any use whatever of its left arm, of which it seemed to be absolutely unaware" (*loc. cit.*, p. 419).

The activity of the cortex is essentially that of sensory discrimination. But in consequence of observations during the war, made in conjunction with Riddoch, Head succeeded in dividing this activity into a series of special functions with autonomy and a very complete reciprocal independence.[2]

First of all, he claims, comes recognition of spatial relations, conditioning the three following processes; the power of appreciating direction and amplitude of movement made passively, which is the most delicate and the most susceptible of change; discrimination between two contacts; and localization of spots touched.

Then follows a graduated appreciation of intensity in tactile excitation, very quickly abolished in cortical lesions.

Finally, recognition of similarity and difference (in the size, shape, weight and texture of objects) becomes individualized.

The three fundamental functions of the cortex would

[1] *Cf.* Turro, "Les origines des représentations de l'espace tactile," II, *Journal de Psychologie*, XVII, 1920, pp. 878-903.

[2] *Cf.* H. Head, "Sensation and the Cerebral Cortex," *Brain*, 1918, XLI, 2, pp. 57-253.—H. Head and G. Riddoch, "Sensory Disturbances in the Hand following Injuries of the Cerebral Cortex," *British Medical Journal*, 1920, II, pp. 782-783.

seem to be separately abolished or preserved in cerebral lesions.

There is nothing astonishing in the fact that in disturbances of perception there may be a predominance of disturbances of the gnosic functions, in the appreciation of contacts, or in spatial representation. But Head's constructions in the course of his interesting experimental analysis have little homogeneity, and he still confuses purely receptive injuries (kinæsthesia giving information on all passive movements) with processes of intellectual identification and associative recognition. He even neglects the incito-associative receptive function of the projection centres of the cortex, and after dealing with discrimination and localization as simple sensations with special conductors, he proceeds to treat them as forms and aspects of a spatial function peculiar to the cortex, going thus from one extreme to the other.

Head is really concerned less with distinct functions than with elementary forms of tactile thought: spatial appreciation, graduation of intensity, and finally, knowledge of the nature of the stimuli.[1] The problem is one of perceptions which give place to more complex identifications, the representation of objects placed at the point of excitation, and the reconstruction of an external environment, with the support of data from the specialized senses.

We are dealing here with types of associative

[1] The recognition of shape—as of the texture of objects—certainly seems to be a cortical perceptive function, and it is impossible to assume with Winkler that impressions of shape are formed in the thalamus, for tactile as well as for visual shape, by combinations of cutaneous and kinæsthetic data—or retinal and kinæsthetic data—and that they are transmitted to the cortex already elaborated; this view is based on observations of astereognosis due to thalamic lesions; but the disturbances in question could have been explained by deficiencies in the elementary data from which the perception of shape is elaborated (*Cf.* Winkler, "A Tumour in the Pulvinar Thalami Optici. A Contribution to the Knowledge of the Vision of Forms," *Folia Neurobiologica*, 1911, V, 7; *Manuel de Neurologie*, I, *Anatomie du système nerveux*, 1918, p. 323).

reaction peculiar to the cortical system,[1] correctly opposed to the unqualified affective reactivity of the thalamus and usefully analysed by Head. But it would be dangerous, on the one hand, to forget that a receptive intercalation of sensory impulses is necessary before this reactivity is possible, and that intercalation may itself be abolished, sometimes unequally according to the various types of cutaneous and deep sensibility; and no less dangerous to derive, from these various types of cortical reaction, new entities with true autonomy and complete independence.

[1] In the general conception which Pavlov has constructed on the basis of his work on the conditioned reflex, he regards as an essential function of the cortex its receptive rôle, which consists in analysing and synthesizing the afferent excitations. ("Die normale Tätigkeit und allgemeine Konstitution der Grosshirnrinde," *Skandivn. Archiv. für Physiologie*, 1923, pp. 32-42).

CHAPTER III

VISUAL RECEPTION

THE influence exercised by visual impressions on the behaviour of the higher mammals is considerable and has greatly facilitated the study of the cortical receptive centres of these impressions by the method of partial extirpation, particularly in that, as contrasted with diffuse sensory impressions, the ablation of the cortical centres involves the complete suppression of total reactions which are manifested in behaviour under the influence of retinal impressions.

Except as regards experiments under unsatisfactory conditions, such as those undertaken to prove a theory by S. I. Franz, there is complete agreement among physiologists.[1] An animal deprived of its occipital areas is really blind: it blunders into obstacles, and does not react, by movements of the eyes, head or body, to diversely localized luminous stimuli, nor does it blink at the sudden approach of the hand.[2]

The pupil, however, reacts to changes in light, and under the sudden influence of a strong light, even without the thermal influence mentioned by Minkowski,

[1] When visual disturbances after occipital extirpation are transitory, it is because the truly receptive portion has not been completely destroyed, as Kurzveil's experiments have long proved ("Beitrag zur Lokalisation der Sehsphäre des Hundes," *Arch. für die ges Physiol.*, 1909, CXXIX, pp. 607-625).

[2] Ablation of one of the occipital areas causes blindness in the hemi-fields of vision of both eyes situated on the opposite side (which corresponds to the two homolateral hemi-retinæ), each retina being in optical connection with the nasal hemi-retina of one eye (which represents two-thirds of the fibres of the corresponding optic nerve) and the temporal hemi-retina of the other.

it can produce a palpebral closing, characteristic of the 'dazzle reflex.'[1]

Apart from these two reflexes, which are dependent on sub-cortical relay stations, all the other motor reflexes produced by ocular impressions disappear in the higher mammals along with the adapted reactions.

It has been possible to determine the visual area in animals, and the projection tracts followed, from the retina to the region of the cortex which adjoins the calcarine fissure and extends deep into the opening

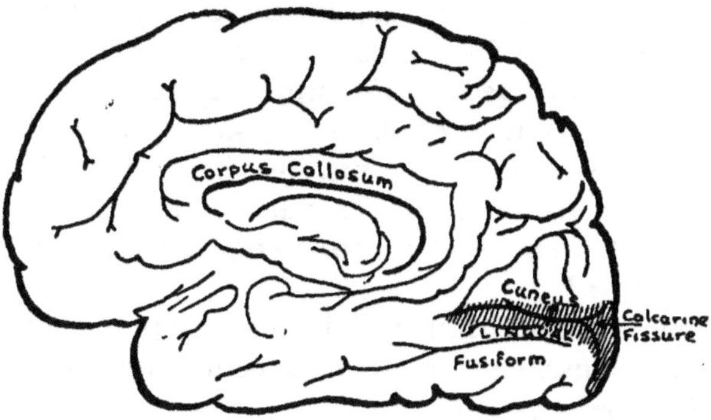

FIG. 12. The striate area of Elliot Smith and Brodmann (shaded) round the calcarine fissure (internal surface of the right hemisphere).

of this fissure. Correspondences can be established, thanks to the degeneration which follows partial lesions, between areas in the sub-cortical relay centres and the surface of the terminal receptive area.[2]

When we turn to the consideration of man, disturbances of vision are sufficiently evident for occipital lesions to have been the object of much anatomical and pathological study; and during the war particularly evidence

[1] *Cf.* Rothmann, "Der Hund ohne Grosshirn," C.R. in *Neurologisches Centralblatt*, 1909, XXVIII, p. 1045.—Dusser de Barenne, *Arch. nėerl de Ph.*, 1919, IV, p. 57.

[2] *Cf.* M. Minkowski, "Zur Physiologie der Sehsphäre," *Pflügers Archiv.* 1911, CXLI, pp. 141-327; "Ueber die Sehrinde und ihre Beziehungen zu den primären optischen Zentren," *Deutsche Zeitschr* f. *Nervenheilk*, 1914, XXXV, p. 420.

was accumulated and remarkable precision was attained in the topography of the retinal projection on the cortex.

1. *Receptive Topography*

Von Monakow assumed that the projection fibres of the retina were scattered in a diffuse manner in the occipital cortex; and his view represented a reaction against the extreme localizing theory.[1]

In opposition to this, Henschen declared in his remarkable work that the retina was projected in some way, point by point, on the surface of the cortex, that the upper edge of the calcarine fissure of one hemisphere corresponded to the upper quadrants of the halves of the retinæ of the same side, and the lower edge to the lower quadrants, the base of the fissure representing the horizontal meridian; and also that the central yellow spot had a special representation in the anterior area.[2]

Though his localization of the macular projection was inexact, Henschen's other statements have received startling confirmation.

Just before the war, in an important thesis, Monbrun[3] made a general review of the literature on quadrantic hemianopsia (54 anatomico-clinical observations), and recorded a series of seven personal observations. He concluded:

that the cortical centre of vision is localized and limited to the calcarine fissure and the adjacent cortex;

[1] C. von Monakow, *Gehirnpathologie*, 2nd Edit., 1901.

[2] *Cf.* Henschen, "La projection de la retine sur la corticalité calcarine," *Semaine médicale*, April 22, 1903. Henschen has recently reminded us of his share, which is too often overlooked, in the discovery of visual localization. "On the Value of the Visual Centre. A Review and a Personal Apology," *Scandinavian Scientific Review*, 1924, III, pp. 10-13).

[3] A Monbrun, *L'Hemianopsie en quadrant*, Paris Thesis, 1914. The principal observations made use of were derived from war cases, and were collected in the Russo-Japanese War by T. Inouye (*Die Sehstörungen bei Schutz erletzungen der korticalen Sehsphäre nach Beobachtungen an Verwandteten der letzten japanichen Kriege*, Leipzig, 1909).

that the optic radiations are divided into two bundles, independent anatomically and physiologically, a superior and an inferior;

that the upper quadrant of the retina corresponds to the superior bundle of the radiations, and is projected on the upper edge of the calcarine area (hemianopsia in the lower quadrant); and inversely;

that the macula is projected on to the extreme posterior part of the calcarine area (hemianopsic macular scotoma);

that the projection is the same for light, form and colour: a partial destruction of the cortex or of the radiations determines a constant, absolute and definite hemianopsic sector.

Returning to the question in the light of the material provided by the war, he shows that all these conclusions have been verified.[1]

In fact, among neurologists such as Pierre Marie and Chatelin, and ophthalmologists such as Morax, in France as well as in England (Gordon Holmes, J. A. Wilson, Riddoch, etc.), Italy (Grignolo,[2] Pari, Trocello, etc.), and Germany (Poppelreuter, Dimmer, Best, etc.), agreement is complete, and the topographical schema may be regarded as well established.

Thanks to an ingenious process by which projectiles which have entered the cerebrum in living patients can be successfully located by means of X-ray photographs in two perpendicular planes, Pierre Marie and Chatelin,[3] on the basis at first of 36 and afterwards of 40 new cases

[1] A. Monbrun, "Les hémianopsies en quadrant et le centre cortical de la vision," *Presse Médicale*, Oct. 22, 1917, p. 607.

[2] There is an extensive but very incomplete bibliography on visual disturbances due to war wounds in Grignolo, "Le lesioni dell' apparato visivo nelle ferite di guerra del cranio," *Giornale della R. Accad. di Med. di Torino*, 1919, LXXXII, Mémoires, pp. 3-98.

[3] Pierre Marie and Chatelin, "Les troubles visuels dus aux lésions des voies optiques intra-cérébrales et de la sphère visuelle corticale dans les blessures du crâne par coup de feu," *Rev. Neur.*, 1915, XXII, pp. 882-925, and *Rev. Neur.*, 1916, XXIII, p. 138.

of visual disturbance due to occipital wounds, were able to establish:

that the cortical centre of vision is localized in the calcarine fissure and in the adjacent cortex (the lower part of the cuneus and the upper part of the lingual lobe);

that the upper quarter of the retina is projected on the upper edge of the calcarine area (hemianopsia in the lower quadrant through cortical destruction);

that a limited lesion of the cortical visual area, on one side, produces a scotoma of a hemianopsic type in each half of the visual field of the opposite side;

that the macula is projected in the posterior part of the area in the neighbourhood of the tip of the occipital lobe.

A little later, W. T. Lister and Gordon Holmes concluded from a study based on a score of observations:

that the upper half of each retina is represented on the dorsal (or upper) part of each visual area, and the lower half on the ventral (or lower) part;

that the centre for macular or central vision is located on the posterior extremities of the visual areas, probably on the edges and lateral surfaces of the occipital lobes.

The portion of each upper quadrant of the retina in the immediate neighbourhood of the fovea, together with the adjacent part of the fovea, has its representation on the upper and posterior part of the visual area in the hemisphere of the same side, and *vice versa.*[1]

In the representation of the peripheral retina—the yellow spot excepted—the projection of the retinal quadrants has long ceased to be a matter of doubt. In each quadrant, the distinct projection of each retinal point has been shown by small scotomata, small blind areas in the two corresponding retinal quadrants, pro-

[1] W. T. Lister and Gordon Holmes, *Proceed. of Roy. Soc. of Medicine of London*, 1916, IX, 4, Sect. of Ophalm., pp. 57-96.

duced by wounds due to minute shell splinters, which destroyed only a minimal zone of the visual area, whose distribution corresponds less to the morphological design

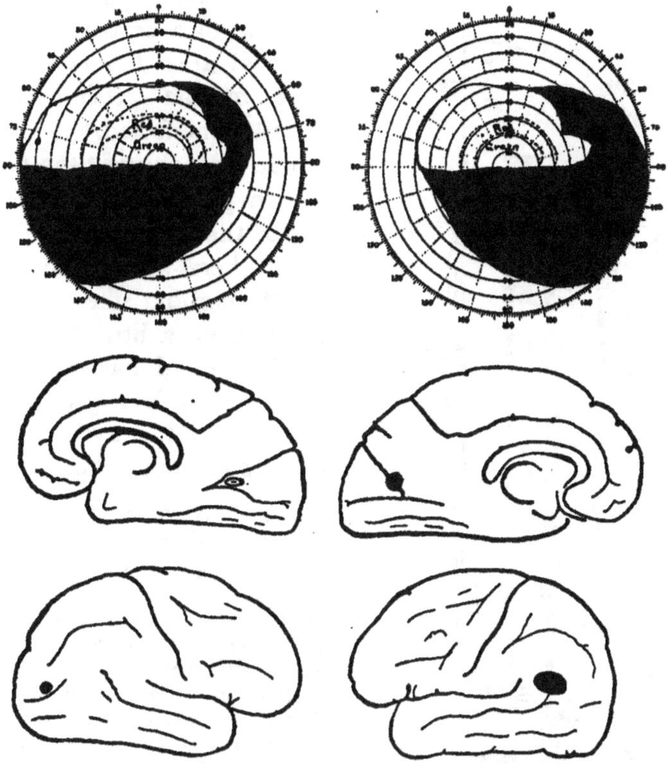

FIG. 13. An observation of horizontal hemianopsia, in the double lower quadrant (the blind region in black), after Gordon Holmes, with diagrams of the lesions affecting the upper part of the striate area in the two hemispheres, whence the blindness in the two upper halves (corresponding to the lower visual fields) of the two retinæ.

of the cortex than to the cyto-architectonic structure (Elliot Smith's *area striata* histologically studied by Brodmann or the so-called area with 8 cellular layers).[1]

[1] We may recall that Brodmann (*Vergleichende Lokalisations—lehre der Grosshirnrinde*, 1909), retaining the fundamental division into 6 layers, distinguishes in the *area striata*: 1, the zonal layer (Cajal's plexiform); 2, the external granular; 3, the pyramidal (small and medium pyramidal); 4, the

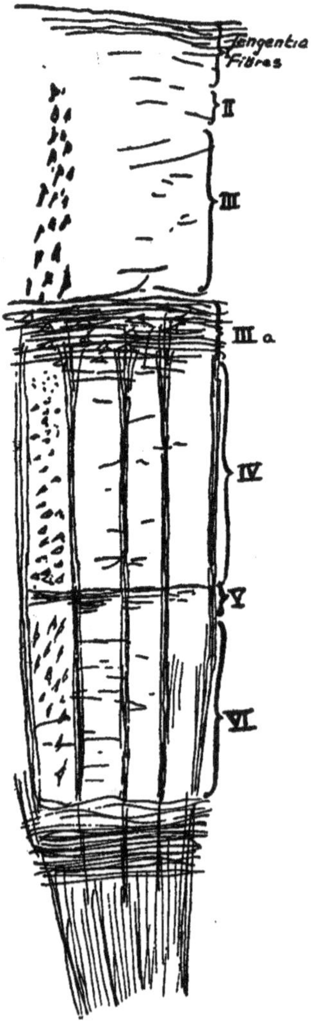

But for the central area of the retina the question is much more controversial: in fact, in complete hemianopsias, seemingly due to a destruction of the visual area of one hemisphere macular vision was generally unaffected.

These facts suggest the following hypotheses: either the fibres of the macula mix with the peripheral fibres and extend throughout the visual area, or even a little beyond (Dejerine, von Monakow, etc.); or each macula is projected as a whole into the two hemispheres, so that macular vision

FIG. 14. Visual cortex (area striata) after Von Monakow.

The great development of the communication fibres is noticeable: in particular, beside the vertical medullary striae, the horizontal strata whose white matter is visible to the naked eye (the strata of Gennari or bundle of Vicq-d'Azyr) at IIIa especially (upper stratum) and at V (lower stratum). The enormous development of layer IV (internal granular with stellate cells) will be noted, and the reduction of the ganglionated layer V (so well-developed in the motor cortex, with the Betz cells).

---

internal granular which is divided into a superficial stratum, an intermediate stratum (the striate stratum of Vicq-d'Azyr or of Gennari, with large stellate cells, characteristic of the visual area), and a deep stratum (small stellate cells); 5, the ganglionated (with large pyramidal cells or Meynert's single cells), and 6, the multiform, divided into an angular stratum (large cells with a curved ascending neurite) and a fusiform stratum (triangular and fusiform cells). In cases of previous blindness of peripheral origin, we note proportionally a considerable reduction in the 4th layer (Bolton).

itself can only be abolished in cortical blindness by double lesion, just as audition disappears only after a double temporal lesion ; or finally the macula is projected in a less vulnerable area, which was located by Inouye, after examination of patients wounded in the Russo-Japanese War, in the posterior part of the occipital lobe (1909).

The existence of hemianopsia with the inclusion of the macula, and, on the other hand, of double hemianopsia with persistence of central vision, of hemimacular scotomata by isolated lesions of the tip of the occipital lobe on one side alone, and finally of double macular scotomata due to lesions of the points of the two occipital lobes, has shown that the last hypothesis was the only true one ; with this reservation, that at the exact centre of the fovea, at the fixation point, there is doubtless a mixing of fibres going towards one or other of the hemispheres, so that the destruction of a single visual area never abolishes vision in this central point. This is analogous to what is established concerning the median line of separation of the innervation of the skin by each hemisphere. And the region of macular projection has been proved to be situated at the tip of the occipital lobe.[1]

The fact that the macular centre occurs in this area, which is situated very low, near the cerebellum and the bulbar level, explains its slight vulnerability, at least in cephalic wounds compatible with survival; and this remains true, although the surface of macular projection be large, especially in relation to the smallness of the

[1] *Cf.* Morax, Moreau and Castelain, "Les différents types d'altération de la vision maculaire dans les lésions traumatiques occipitales," *Annales d'Oculistique*, 1919, CLVI, pp. 1-24.—V. Morax, "Discussion des hypothèses faites sur les connexions corticales des faisceaux maculaires," *Ibid.*, pp. 25-35. —B. Bramwell, J. Bolton, and W. Robinson, "Bilateral Lesion of the Occipital Lobes with Retention of Macular as distinct from Panoramic Vision," *Brain*, 1915, XXXVIII, pp. 447-472 (and Bramwell, *Edinburgh Medical Journal*, 1915, XV, pp. 4-18).—F. Dimmer, "Zwei Falle von Schussverletzungen der centralen Seebahnen," *Wien. Kl. Woch.*, 1915, XXVIII, pp. 519-524;—Trocello. *Ann. di Med. Navale*, 1920, XXVI, 1; etc.

corresponding retinal surface, because of the density of the distinct receptive elements in the central area of vision.

Basing his opinions in large measure on his personal observations, Gordon Holmes[1] succeeded in locating on the *area striata*, assuming the edges of the calcarine fissure to be turned back to disclose the cortex covering

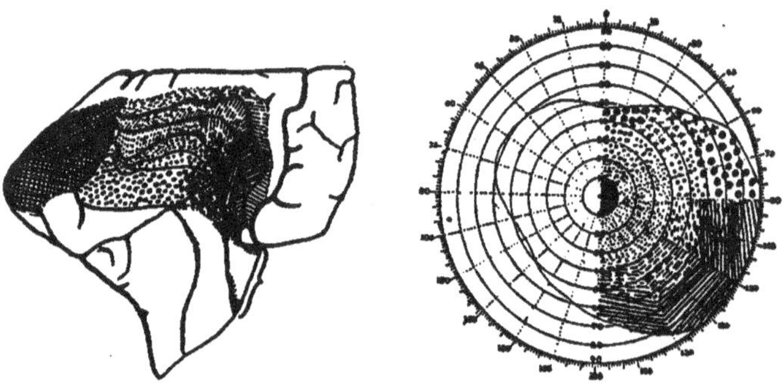

Fig. 15. Diagram of the projection of the visual field (and consequently of the retinal surface) upon the area striata, after Gordon Holmes.

The various regions of the field are repeated on the section of the cortex, so that it can be seen when the edges of the calcarine fissure are drawn back. Above the bottom of the fissure are projected the fields of the lower half (corresponding to the upper retinal quadrant); in front are the most peripheral fields; the macula is represented behind, at the tip of the occipital lobe, with its proper divisions.

its walls, the peripheral and macular sectors of the retinæ. The very possibility of this schematization shows how much our knowledge of the receptive topography of visual impressions has increased in consequence of the great number of occipital war-lesions, and how fully the idea of a point by point representation of the peripheral sensory surface on the cerebral cortex has been verified.

1 Gordon Holmes, "Disturbances of Vision by Cerebral Lesions," *British Journal of Opthalmology*, 1918, II, pp. 353-384.

2. *Relations of the Various Forms of Visual Impression*

Unlike smell, vision covers more than one category of sensations; we distinguish crude sensations of light, delicate impressions of chromatic shade, and discrimination of form, which is effected especially by macular vision.

As a matter of fact, elementary vision of form is essentially connected with the spatial discrimination of unequally excited retinal points and with distinctions between neighbouring areas of light and shade. It therefore involves a perceptive process, with graduated reactions differing specifically, brought into play by adjacent neurones.

This is a function necessarily more vulnerable than the crude reaction to a luminous stimulus perceived *in toto*, and appreciated in an unqualified way as regards intensity, allowing only a vague localization, controlled by the hemisphere which is excited.

And, in fact, in partial injuries, perception of light in the hemianopsic field may be intact, while perception of form, which is normally vague in the peripheral parts of the field, is completely abolished. This is what Bard meant when he said that hemiamblyopia is a weaker form of hemianopsia, the crude vision of light being the *ultimum moriens.*[1]

The fact is analogous to that established in injuries of the cortical sensory area, where a slight raising of the absolute threshold of tactile excitation accompanies a considerable rise of the differential threshold and of the threshold of discrimination, and noticeable errors in localization result.

But chromatic reception is even more vulnerable than perceptive functioning, which implies the integrity of the associational neurones and the isolated reception of

[1] The threshold of luminous vision in a case of hemianopsia through an occipital wound, which came under my notice, was only eight times as high on the practically blind side as on the intact side. But the differential threshold could not be measured, and there was no impression of form.

each of the impulses conducted by the corresponding association paths, without that diffusion which results when the myelin sheaths which isolate the conducting fibres are destroyed. Though Bard regarded hemianopsia as the first stage of cortical injury, then hemiachromatopsia and finally absolute hemiamblyopia, a disturbance, however slight, when it can be discovered produces hemiachromatopsia, that is to say, blindness to colour, almost always total, though sometimes only partial, as in one of Grignolo's cases, even when perception of form persists. Hemiastereopsia[1] is a still more serious disorder, hemiaphotopsia constituting complete blindness of the homologous hemi-retinæ.[2]

According to certain writers, we should distinguish yet another order of visual sensations, the loss of which represents an intermediate stage between astereopsia and aphotopsia, namely, sensations of movement. The crude perception of light and movement (a white test object against a black background or a black one against a luminous background) appear in the first stage of the recovery of vision after cortical blindness due to cranial injury in the occipital area, according to G. Riddoch.[3] Head has also noted a case of partial hemianopsia in which the impossibility of defining stationary objects existed together with a certain appreciation of movement.[4] Finally, Poppelreuter adds the sensation of

[1] *Cf.* H. Piéron, "Des degrés de l'hémianopsie corticale: L'hémiastéréopsie," *C. R. Société de Biologie*, 1916, LXXIX. p. 1055.

[2] Normally the achromatopsia may be a lasting residue of a complete hemianopsia, or it may appear in a transient fashion during functional recovery (Pierre Marie and Chatelin, and Monbrun). Thus we have hemiachromatopsic scotomata which may exist alone or with hemianopsic scotomata. When accentuation or regression occurs (compressive sanguinary diffusions with subsequent slow reabsorption, for example) we can see disturbances of the three forms of vision succeeding one another in the same order (*cf.* Morax. "L'hémianopsie par contusion du crâne," *Annales d'Oculistique*, 1918, CLVIII, pp. 112-121—Monbrun, "Le centre cortical de la vision," *Archives d'Ophtalmologie*, 1919, XXXVI, 11).

[3] "Dissociation of Visual Perceptions due to Occipital Injuries, with especial Reference to Appreciation of Movement," *Brain*, 1917, XL, pp. 15-17.

[4] *Proceedings of the Roy. Soc. of Medicine*, 1918, Sect. of Neurology, p. 27.

movement to the sensations of brightness and colour and acuteness of discrimination.[1] He noted that an object which is invisible when motionless will be seen if it is moved.

But this idea of a specific sensation of movement, maintained by Riddoch in particular, cannot be accepted: it is a normal and well-known fact that an object is more easily seen by the peripheral retina when it is in motion than when it is at rest; the fact that it appears and disappears in its place will also facilitate vision. This is a phenomenon of orientation of the attention and a lowering of the threshold by specific reinforcement (or diminution of an inhibitory influence, or even both).

On the other hand, appreciation of movement is more delicate, especially in peripheral vision, than appreciation of extensity, and consequently of form; this is also a normal well-known fact, analogous to that of a much more exact discrimination between successive than simultaneous contacts, by cutaneous sensibility.

Movement reinforces photopsia or stereopsia, and thus allows us to demonstrate more readily the existence of one of these forms of vision when they are considerably injured. But it does not constitute an elementary specific retinal sensation, which is very difficult to conceive. The appreciation of movement is a perception based on elementary local impressions.

The fact remains that though efforts have long been made to locate a special centre[2] for colour-vision which is superposed on light-vision, from which it is sharply distinguished, in the cortical projection of the retina, as the tactile, thermal, or kinæsthetic sensibilities are superposed in the cortical projection of the cutaneous surface, it has invariably proved to be extremely vulner-

1 Walther Poppelreuter, *Die psychischen Schädigungen durch Kopfschuss im Kriege*, I, 1917.

2 Willbrand, for example, had assumed three distinct centres for luminous, chromatic and spatial vision. He was subsequently forced to admit the unity of the visual centre which to-day is no longer questioned.

able in contradistinction to the different cutaneous sensations.

The observation by Lenz of a microscopic alteration of one only of the eight extraordinarily rich cellular layers[1] which characterize the *area striata* of Elliot Smith and Brodmann, the area of visual reception, in conjunction with the presumptive existence of a pure hemiachromatopsia might suggest in this relatively superficial layer of cells, specific chromatic neurones (the upper pyramidal cells).

But this susceptibility cannot be explained by a greater vulnerability of the layer of cells controlling chromatic sensory reactions. In fact, cerebral compression by tumours involving functional disturbances may produce hemiachromatopsias which disappear after decompression;[2] in partial injuries even of the optic tracts and of the chiasma, hemiachromatopsia is often the first phenomenon to occur.[3]

In order to explain this we must take into account the way in which a chromatic sensation can be evoked in a given point of the retina. The light exciting this point arouses a sensation of brightness of graduated intensity, endowed with a local signature linked with the corresponding connecting neurone of the cortex,[4] and has its

[1] The divisions vary considerably with different writers. The relation between them has been explained by Bonne in his excellent work on the cerebral cortex (Part II), published by the *Revue gén d'Histologie*, 1910, III 12, p. 246.

[2] P. Bordley and H. Cushing, "Alterations in the Colour Fields in Cases of Brain Tumour," *Arch. of Ophthalmology*, 1909, XXXVIII, pp. 451-462.

[3] *Cf.* Pierre Marie and Chatelin, "Les troubles visuels consécutifs aux blessures des voies optiques centrales et de la sphère visuelle corticale: hémianopsies en quadrant supérieur; Hémiachromatopsies," *Revue Neurologique*, 1916, XXIII, p. 138.

[4] The 'corresponding' points of the two hemi-retinæ, for which, in binocular vision, there is a single spatial impression, end in different neurones and not in a single neurone (*cf.* Minkowski, "Sur la terminaison et la représentation centrale des fibres croisées et directes des nerfs optiques," "Contribution à l'anatomie et à la physiologie de la vision binoculaire," Congrès de Physiologie de Paris, 1920, *Arch. suisses de Neurol.* et de Psych., II and III; "Sur les conditions anatomiques de la vision binoculaire dans les voies optiques centrales," *Encéphale*, 1922, II, 65-96). But these neurones which must be

own associative circuits, governing especially certain fixed ocular reflexes (the movement of the eye assuring centro-foveal fixation, for example, for a peripheral point). If the light is coloured, it is further necessary that the nervous impulse coming from the excited retinal receptive cone, in the case of a punctiform luminous foreground, shall be able to secure the activation of a specific neurone for the degree of light (and the number of perceptible gradations—apart from variations in brightness and saturation, that is to say, in the relation between the chromatic impression and the impression of brightness—is considerable, between 50 and 150, at any rate for the central points).

For this reason the projection fibre of this cone, in connection with the series of chromatic neurones—each with its local specificity which is a function of this connection—must act at a single touch of this keyboard according to the length of the dominant wave of the luminous excitation. These phenomena of syntonization are doubtless due, as we shall see later, to the peculiar chronaxic coefficients of these neurones and to the modification of the nervous impulse correlative to the variations of the length of the predominant wave. In fact, though we are not at present able to give an account of the mechanism of peripheral transformation, we know that the negative retinal variation, which gives us a sort of translation of the nervous impules itself, changes its form according to the colour of the light (perhaps by a combination resulting from two or three elementary processes).

This delicate evocation of chromatic tones requires—even more than the changing of circuits for the minimal variations in intensity required by the graduated sensi-

associated, and which are integrated in the same associative and reflex circuits, possess for that very reason a single local specificity. An experimental dissociation, as the facts have shown, can cause the neurones of these corresponding points to acquire a different local specificity (strabismus) and can make two other neurones associate with them in common circuits giving them the same local sign.

bility which appears in the determination of the differential thresholds—the complete integrity of the neurones transmitting the impulses, and especially the syntonized neurones of the chromatic keyboard, for the proper coefficient of the neurone is modified by the slightest injury which it undergoes. A functional disturbance, without complete destruction, deranges and easily incapacitates the chromatic keyboard, which represents not so much an individualized mode of sensibility (as hot or cold in relation to touch) as a different mode of response to certain luminous excitations.

3. *Perceptive Functions and Visual Co-ordination*

The calcarine area of the *area striata* is traditionally known as the 'centre of vision.' But the expression is incorrect. The act of vision does not occur entirely in this receptive station; it involves the operation of the associative circuits which not only traverse the occipital lobe, but sometimes extend as far as the other pole of the brain. Lesions at various points may be shown by disturbances of visual function, though we are then, of course, no longer concerned with disturbances of elementary reception.

In certain cases, special centres for definite visual functions have been assumed; for example, it has often been supposed that there is a centre where visual memories would be stored, a centre of perception where visual ideas would be elaborated, etc.

Von Monakow has rightly opposed such views; memory should be regarded as a dynamic function and not as a storehouse of images. In his opinion, the mnemonic function extends over a large area. And it is certain that disturbances of visual evocation accompany occipital lesions even beyond the calcarine area. On the other hand, when he assumes that the evocation of visual representations remains possible, as a general function, in spite of the destruction of the receptive station, he is allowing himself to fall into the same error which made him deny the topographical representation of the retina on the *area striata.*

The evocation of a visual image implies activation in an associative circuit necessarily including specific connecting neurones in the receptive station. When these are destroyed it is impossible to evoke sensations. And the absence of visual representations in complete cortical blindness among adults, apart from blindness through retinal injury or interruption of the optic tracts, is an established fact. Many instances are cited where hallucinations are produced in the blind part of the field in cerebral hemianopsia; but in no case has an autopsy revealed a complete cortical destruction of the *area striata.* If the lesion interrupts, in the subjacent white matter, the incoming tracts or even the first neurones of the lower cortical layers,[1] without damaging the stellate cells of the median layers, which are characteristic of the visual area and should constitute the specific connecting neurones,[2] hallucinations clearly remain possible. If, on the other hand, the cortical lesion prevents the functioning of the specific neurones, and even if a certain crude luminous vision persists, as in a case I observed, these hallucinations are only produced in the part of the field where vision is preserved.[3]

[1] After section of the optic tracts there is a correlative degeneration of the polymorphous cells of the last cortical layer and of the solitary cells of layer V of Brodmann (von Monakow).

[2] Ramon y Cajal places the "anatomical seat of sensation" in the layer of the large stellate cells: supposing that the axone of these large cells conducts "the principal optical excitation, which is to be registered in the form of memories or optical images" (*Studien über die Hirnrinde,* 1900, "Die Sehrinde," p. 71). Rouvière emphasizes the fact that these cells, about which ramify the prolongations of the small pyramidal cells, the granules, are not influenced by the fibres of the superficial layer (Cajal's plexiform layer).

[3] On the subject of hemianopsic hallucinations, see: Wilfred Harris, "Hemianopia, with Especial Reference to its Transient Varieties," *Brain,* 1897, XX, pp. 308-364;—H. Roger and J. Reboul-Lachaux, "Le syndrome excito-visuel du champ aveugle des hémianopsiques," *L'Encéphale,* 1921, XVI,

The sensation of blackness in the blind part of the field no longer appears when hemianopsia is due to cortical destruction : this sensation is no more possible than the others (for it is that of a very slight brightness appearing by contrast). Hemianopsic blindness of cortical origin is not recognized, and wounded men are astonished at the awkwardness which makes them blunder into obstacles, always on their blind side; their hemianopsia has to be explained to them.[1]

Von Monakow[2] even cites the case of a patient blinded by double occipital destruction, who was able to imagine a wax taper, though he could not give its characteristics. But to attach importance to such a remark[3] is to overlook the difficulty of distinguishing in many cases between true visual memory, with representation of forms by light and shade, and memory by simple ocular kinæsthesia, which gives a very satisfying representation of form, and one which is regarded as visual.

If the memory of ocular kinæsthesia is preserved, and particularly if movements of the eyes are still possible, we imagine that we are calling up visual

pp. 573-579. In one of Kinnier Wilson's cases, micropsic hallucinations appeared in the hemianopsic field, but only after recovery of vision, which was destroyed as the result of an occipital fracture (*Lancet*, 1917, 2, CXCIII, p. 1).

[1] Dufour has discussed very carefully this question of the distinction (J. Müller, de Graefe) between 'Schwarzsehen' and 'Nichtssehen' ("Sur la vision nulle dans l'hémianopsie," *Revue médicale de la Suisse romande*, 1889, 9th year, VIII, pp. 445-451). Such a difference in visual behaviour has also been recently considered by Fuchs ("Untersuchungen über das Sehen der Hemianopiker und Hemiamblyopiker," *Zeitschr. für Psychologie*, 1921, LXXXVI, pp. 1-143).

[2] *Cf.* Von Monakow, "Ueber den gegenwartigen Stand . . . ," *Ergebnisse der Physiologie*, 1904, III (II), p. 118.

[3] Experimental analysis of the memory of forms insusceptible of symbolic schematization has convinced me of the great importance of ocular kinæsthesia and the small part played by visualization in nearly all individuals, with the general illusion of really visual representations, a very strong illusion, especially when symbolic and verbal schematization is possible. Ideas which are substituted for visual representation, and play the same part, are easily mistaken for it (*cf.* H. Piéron, "Recherches comparatives sur la mémoire des formes et celle des chiffres," *Année Psychologique*, 1921, XXI, pp. 119-148).

memories, for many people, in ordinary circumstances, have no true visual representation other than kinæsthetic.

The specific neurones necessary for sensation are also necessary for the associative reawakening of that sensation, which is called the image—a dynamic process and not a photographic negative resting miraculously in the nervous substance, where some subtle spirit might go to consult it.

But these are probably not sufficient; an impulse of peripheral origin, operating certain notes of the keyboard formed by the specific neurones, could not by this act alone produce a sensation, which is a psychical phenomenon; this results from an excitation of the associative area by the specific connecting neurones; reception begins at the level of the calcarine area with its rich and varied group of cells, but is completed in wide and numerous circuits.

While the tracts which directly produce certain reflexes apparently issue from the deep layers of the cortex—and further knowledge of these, as we shall see, may provide us with more detailed information—from the superficial layer formed by a network of associative fibres issue the inciting impulses of the neighbouring relay neurones, which themselves enter into connection with all the cerebral areas, auditory, tactile, kinæsthetic, incito-motor, etc.

One of the influences arising from a sudden excitation will constitute the reaction of attention, with the inhibitions it involves, the importance of which in the operation of vision—binocular vision especially—is well known. This reaction of attention, which, as Head has shown, is very much weakened in cortical injuries of the sensory area, is also very easily disturbed[1] in

[1] The disorder in question seems sometimes to have been the only manifestation of the occipital injury, in the cases observed by Gordon Holmes (*Brit. J. of Opht.*, II, 1918, p. 353). It is, of course, not a matter of general weakening of attention, but of an isolated loss of attentive capacity for a certain order of stimuli.

occipital lesions, as Gordon Holmes, Poppelreuter, and Wilhelm Fuchs, each from his particular angle, have also noticed. In an area where the perception of darkness or of light appearing suddenly is possible, when no other object is visible to the eye, nothing may be perceived when another object appears in a normal part of the field: when there are two rival reactions of attention, each tending to provoke the inhibition of other circuits of perception by means of the excitation of another group of connecting neurones, the reaction of the normal cortical area will so predominate that the excitation of the other produces no conscious effects. When the functions are normal there will be a much greater intensity of a peripheral excitation in one field which will annul the psychical effect of a peripheral excitation of the opposite field; reciprocal suppressive inhibition in binocular vision is an ordinary occurrence.

Thus the nervous impulses concerned in vision issue from the connecting neurones and irradiate through the entire brain. But it is certain that a lesion will most easily injure the association paths of visual thought at the approaches to the receptive station. And, as a matter of fact, this function is found to be selectively injured in occipital lesions which leave the calcarine area untouched.

But disturbances of this form of thought may appear in consequence of lesions which, though always localized to some extent, are relatively distant from the receptive area, indicating an interruption of certain intercortical connections of a systematic character.

In so-called psychical blindness, or generalized visual agnosia, there is still vision of objects,[1] general reactions and reflexes left intact, but their associative utilization is no longer possible; objects are no longer recog-

[1] In the most elementary case there is stereoagnosia (or an astereognosis), in the sense that even the recognition of simple forms no longer occurs; it is characteristic only when macular vision is preserved (distinct perception of form being possible only at the centre of the retina).

nized by sight, though still recognized by touch or hearing.[1]

Limited visual agnosias are found, for example, in the form of certain asymbolias: the significance of simple visual signs is no longer understood; cards, flags, etc., are no longer specifically recognized. An ace of clubs might still be recognized as a card, but its particular character, value or use would be unknown. This asymbolia may be generalized or limited, for example, to printed or written signs (verbal agnosia or verbal blindness), and even to certain of these signs, so that only numbers may be misunderstood, or, on the other hand, only numbers may be understood. In order to give an account of these partial disturbances, we must introduce the idea of a co-ordinating centre, that is to say, a systematic grouping of the connecting neurones, which intervene in the associative circuits of certain forms of thought, of symbolic thought in particular, and form an essential stage.

A more detailed examination of this idea of co-ordination will be undertaken in connection with language in general, which involves an important visual component.

[1] F. Best has specially examined, in cases of cranial lesion, disorders of the higher visual functions, which he classes as optico-stereometric disturbances (parietal calcarine region), optico-phasic (temporal region), optico-gnostic (convexity of the occipital lobe), optico-motor, etc. (*Neurol. Centralblatt.*, 1920, p. 290. *Cf.* also Best, "Hemianopsie und Seelindblindheit bei Hirnverletzungen," *Grafe's Archiv.*, 1917, XCIII, H. 1).

CHAPTER IV

INDIRECT RECEPTION

SPATIAL PERCEPTION AND SPATIAL REFLEXES

THE excitation of a receptive apparatus when transmitted to the cortical area produces there a specific associative reaction, ensuring identification and the corresponding sensory perception. Sometimes what reaches this association area is the after-effect of an excitation in direct relation with the thalamus and the affective area: as happens in the case of certain 'pains,' such as burning. Or the specific excitation may be accompanied by an awareness of the affective reverberation (pricking). The organic impressions of cœnæsthesia, pleasures and pains especially, are specific excitations of the affective centres, and penetrate into associative 'knowledge' only through their means.

Certain of these organic impressions which reach the higher centres will at times be adequate only in the degree in which they have previously aroused reflexes in more primitive centres. Thus hunger may indeed be an impression produced by a certain state of various organs, but it will reach the affective area—and *a fortiori* the associative—only through movements of the stomach which have been previously produced, and which may also occur automatically in accordance with a regular rhythm. Thirst is due to a dehydration of the blood and the tissues, but it is perceived only when a reflex inhibition of salivation, a result of this dehydration, produces a perceptible dryness of the throat which brings into operation the appetitive tendencies, the desire to drink, and arouses specifically directed associations.

There are in reality numerous sensations which, from the point of view of 'knowledge,' in our system of representations, have a direct objective significance, though they are actually due to a secondary effect of primitive excitations.

It is not enough to establish the existence of a specialized receptive organ on the one hand, and of sensations corresponding to the excitation of this organ on the other, in order to conclude that it is the latter which is directly transmitted to the association area to enable a specific awareness to arise there.

Thus the excitation of the semicircular canals, which involves indispensable equilibration reflexes, does not seem capable of directly producing associative reactions, sensations and perceptions: and, in fact, there is no tract uniting the nuclei of the vestibular nerve with the cerebral cortex. Furthermore, the sensations of rotation, and in particular the subsequent post-rotary sensations, are unquestionably connected with the excitation of the horizontal canals: they give the impression of a rotation of the body towards the right or towards the left, when the eyes are closed, and of a rotation of external objects in the opposite direction when the eyes are open.

In reality, these sensations, these associative reactions which give the knowledge of right and left, are produced by the perception of ocular movements accompanying and following the rotation (rotary and post-rotary nystagmus); the slow reflex displacement of the eye (such as occurs in rotation when the eye follows an object), being perceived not as actual movement but as the rotation of objects in this direction, or as a rotation of the body—in the absence of vision of objects—in the opposite direction.

The threshold of the ocular reflex is, in fact, lower

than the threshold of the sensation;[1] the duration of the apparent movement is connected with that of the nystagmus, being a little shorter;[2] and finally the experiments of Barany and Holt[3] have shown that the inhibition of ocular movements involves the suppression of rotary and post-rotary sensations.

From a long and careful study of nystagmic phenomena, Brabant[4] deduces the following results, which are in full agreement with the above: whenever there is a sensation of movement there is nystagmus; when there is an impression of immobility, the equilibrium of the eyeballs is complete; the direction, rapidity and amplitude of the movement perceived depend on the direction, rapidity and duration of the nystagmic movements. When a suggestion of rotation occurs, ocular movements take place first and it is only later that the subject is aware of rotatory impression.

Though of more complex origin, impressions of displacement and of inclination also seem to be linked with reflex movements; and in a general way we may say with the majority of physiologists, that these spatial data derive from the perception of the reflexes of equilibration whether of labyrinthine origin or not.

For even when we can receive direct sensations, from 'exteroceptor' peripheral organs, when these furnish

[1] *Cf.* E. Buys "Contribution a l'étude du nystagmus de la rotation," *C. R. Soc. de Biologie*, 1920, LXXXIII, p. 1234. The threshold of the sensation corresponds to an angular acceleration of 1°·8 to 2° per second, the threshold of the nystagmic movement to an acceleration of 0°· 8.

[2] *Cf.* Coleman R. Griffith, "The Organic Effects of Repeated Bodily Rotation. An Experimental Study of Dizziness," *J. of Exper-Psychol.*, III, 1, 2, 1920, pp. 15-46 and pp. 87-125. In attempts at the inhibition of ocular movement, the duration of the post-rotary nystagmus and likewise that of the subsequent sensation of rotation is diminished.

[3] *Cf.* R. Barany, "Untersuchungen über den vom Vestibularapparat des Ohres reflektorisch augelösten rhytmischen Nystagmus und seine Begleiterscheinungen," *Monatschrift für Ohrenheilkunde*, XL, 1906, pp. 193-197.—E. B. Holt, "Eye-movements during Dizziness," *Harvard Psychol. Studies*, II, 1906, pp. 57-66; "On Ocular Nystagmus and the Localization of Sensory Data during Dizziness," *Psychological Review*, XVI, 1909, pp. 377-398.

[4] V. G. Brabant, "Nouvelles recherches sur la nystagmus et le sens de l'équilibre," *Archives médicales belges*, 1921, 4th year, 4, pp. 257-324.

spatial perceptions, closely intermingled with sensations and thus appearing to be immediate data, it seems that they can do so only in the degree in which appropriate reactions are aroused, the knowledge of which—by means of the 'proprioceptor' organs—will assume the appearance of direct spatial exteroceptive data.

The reactions thus produced by the specific spatial impressions may, moreover, originate at different levels; they may either be elementary reflexes, in circuits limited to the lower levels of the nervous system, or late and complex reflexes, the connecting neurones of which are situated in the higher centres and in the cortex itself.

In the latter case, it may perhaps be suggested that these reflexes are only automatized associative reactions, acquired during the life of the individual by experience and by trial and error; but there are also congenital reflexes in the cortical area, and though it is indisputable that the intellectual idea of space implies a personal acquisition—peculiarly aided, we may add, by ancestral experience socially transmitted and symbolized by language—the fact remains that this idea in its elementary form can originate from sensory data produced by specific congenital reactions, so that there is some justification for a physiological 'nativism.'

Certainly the spatial location of a sensory excitant appears to be a gradual empirical acquisition. But though the local sign of a sensation does not intellectually gain value and spatial significance until after repeated experiences, it is none the less true that the location of the stimulus involves, in consequence of congenital nervous connections, a certain specificity in the reflex responses that this stimulus can arouse.

The 'acid' reflex in the decerebrate frog and the scratch reflex in the spinal dog imply a fairly exact localization.

Is there still a reflex cutaneous localization in man? There is undoubtedly a local relation between the cutaneous excitation and the reflex response: the plantar stimulation of new-borns, which involves, in addition to the extension of the toes, a retraction of the lower limb concerned, certainly implies a specifically localized influence; and movements of defence adapted to the region stimulated have been established even among anencephalics during the brief period of their survival.[1]

Further: according to an observation of van Woerkom's on a child of four affected with meningo-encephalitis,[2] the excitation of the skin of the foot aroused, besides the retraction of the lower limb, a reflex movement of the hand approaching the place touched and making a vigorous gesture of repulse; and in various meningitic syndromes, Guillain and Barré have noticed a localizing reflex which appears in a similar form:[3] the pinching of the skin of the foot or the leg produced a complex movement in the opposite lower limb, in the course of which the knee was bent and the foot was drawn up to scratch the stimulated region with the heel.

In coma, with abolition of all mental life, movements of defence adapted to the seat of a strong stimulus are found even in hemiplegic patients.

The existence of a reflex localization has suggested that there may be disagreement between the capacity for spatial representation of a cutaneous contact with a description and the capacity for finding with the finger the point stimulated, by itching, for example; this latter process being of a reflex character, in that it represents the operation of a congenital mechanism or an acquired automatism.

Thus a patient with a cerebral injury in the occipital area, who was studied by Goldstein and Gelb, was able to locate, by spasmodic reflex movements, a contact

[1] *Cf.* Vaschide and Vurpas, "La vie biologique d'un anencéphale." *Revue générale des Sciences*, April 30, 1901, p. 373.

[2] Van Woerkom, "Sur les réactions musculaires d'ordre affectif," *Archives suisses de Neurologie et de Psychiatrie*, 1921, VIII, 1.

[3] Guillain and Barré, "Les réflexes de défense vrais au cours des syndromes méningés," *Bull. et. Mém. de la Soc. Méd. des Hopitaux*, 1916.

spot on the skin, though he had no idea of the location of the stimulation.

The authors concluded from this that tactile space does not exist.[1] Their results at least indicated that in this case the spatial schema of the body implied a co-ordinated appeal to the data of sight, and that when this connection was lacking 'spatial thought' was affected; though a new spatial thought, fundamentally tactile, could doubtless arise, thanks to the preservation of the specific reactions.

The reflex origin of auditory spatial data seems even clearer.

The perception of the direction of a source of sound only occurs in virtue of an associative reaction produced by a reflex movement of the head and the eyes in that direction, and also of the vestibule of the ears among certain animals. Localization, indeed, seems congenital and perhaps infra-cortical, by association with the auditory relay centres, at the level of the corpora quadrigemina, with the head-turning and eye-turning co-ordination centres.[2]

For low sounds, a sufficiently accurate localization is ensured by the difference in phase of the vibratory movements of the tympanic membrane in the ears (provided the length of the wave distinctly exceeds the distance between the tympana). But this difference of phase cannot itself involve associative reactions or perceptive knowledge: it arouses reflexes carefully adapted to the value of the difference; and these reflexes in their turn produce impressions of direction, which were sufficiently precise to allow aeroplanes to be located at night during the war.

[1] K. Goldstein and A. Gelb, "Ueber den Einfluss des vollständigen Verlustes des optischen Vorstellungsvermögens auf das taktile Erkennen," *Zeitschr. für Psychologie*, LXXXIII, 1-2.

[2] Reactions of localization to noises have been noticed in decerebrate mammals, in the cat, for example, but not in all cases. Dusser de Barenne does not believe that the seat of these reactions can at present be fixed with certainty.

In researches based on introspective data, Halverson [1] has shown that localization occurs in a visually schematized arc where a tonal image (visual, auditory, kinæsthetic, or tactile image) is located under the influence of an eye-movement whether actually performed or imagined.

For noises or shrill sounds there are differences in intensity at the level of the ears which give, though with much less precision, the idea of direction, an idea that seems to be immediate because the difference in intensity is not perceived as such. And the orientation of the source occurs even when differences in intensity are too weak to be perceptible in themselves and below the differential threshold of the sensation. Here also the differential threshold of the reflex is more delicate, and it is the perception of the localizing reflex which furnishes the idea of space,[2] a reflex involving primarily movements of ocular exploration,[3] while lateralization always appears as due to the exclusive excitation of one ear.

As distinguished from the factor of phase difference, the ratio of sound intensities gives results which as a

[1] Halverson, "Binaural Localization of Tones," *Am. Journal of Psychology*, 1922, XXXIII, pp. 178-212.

[2] By placing an individual at an unequal distance from two identical and synchronous sources of sound, we produce in him the impression of a single source localized at a point in space which depends on the difference, at the level of the ears, in the combination of both trains of waves. This corresponds at the same time to a difference in phase and a difference in intensity. Now, if we modify the frequency of the sound of the sources, and consequently the wave-length, we change the combination and the variation is perceived as an apparent displacement of the imaginary source before it is perceived as a tonal modification. Thus the differential threshold of localization is much more delicate than those of pitch, intensity, and, as we shall see, succession (*cf.* C. E. Seashore, "Wave Phase in the Open-air Localization of Sound," *Psychol. Monographs*, 1922, XXXI, 1, pp. 1-6).

[3] This is the hypothesis of ocular movements suggested by Matsumoto and favoured by Hocart and McDougall, who have shown that the threshold of differentiation in the localization of sound corresponds to a difference of intensity which is less than a third of the differential threshold of perceptions of intensity ("Some Data for a Theory of Auditory Perception of Direction," *British Journal of Psychology*, 1908, II, p. 386).

whole follow Weber's[1] law, showing the slight sensibility of this process; and this is in agreement with the general data of the far less rapid increase of organic reactions in comparison with the increase of *intensities* of excitation that provoke these reactions. When we cause the difference in intensity and the dyschronism to act in the opposite direction (Pérot), the two influences can be compensated, but as that of the dyschronism is predominant, the other must be greatly accentuated.

Finally, for noises of short duration the perception of laterality may be conditioned by the interval which elapses between the moment when the wave enters one ear and that at which it enters the other, an interval notably below the threshold of duration perceptible as such, as Aggazzotti[2] has established, by eliminating any influence of intensity (the thresholds of lateralization being able to sink to 4° and to three hundred-thousandths of a second); but localization is extremely crude (errors amounting to as much as 110°) and practically non-existent. The researches of Pérot[3] are in agreement with those of Aggazzotti.

The recognition of direction, to the right or left of the source, appears to be immediate. In this case it seems as if one ear only is affected, as if the impression reaching the other were inhibited by the first. This impression may arise from a difference in time of impact or a difference of intensity, without our being able to distinguish its origin. We obtain thus an

[1] *Cf.* G. W. Stewart and O. Hovda, "The Intensity Factor in Binaural Localization: an Extension of Weber's Law," *Psychological Review*, 1918, XXV, p. 242.

[2] A. Aggazzotti, "Sulla percezione della direzione del suono," *Archivio di Fisiologia*, 1921, XIX, 1 pp. 33-46.

[3] A. Pérot, "Sur la sensation d'orientation dans l'audition naturelle," *Journal de Physique et le Radium*, 1921, IV, pp. 97-106. For a noise Pérot finds a lateralization corresponding to a difference in time of eight hundred-thousandths of a second, which is quite the same order of magnitude as that of Aggazzotti. Pérot has also studied the influence of differences in intensity, and that of differences of phase for pure sounds, but has confused it with that of differences in times of access of sounds.

impression of lateralization connected with the ocular reaction, but not a precise apparent direction.[1]

It is concerning visual localization that the most frequent and keenest controversy has arisen between those who assume that local retinal signs or binocular separation [2] are acquired by experience, and those who hold that pre-established ideas allow the immediate utilization of local retinal impressions. But here again we must not forget the existence of localizing reflexes which, although they require cortical intervention, seem none the less to be congenitally determined. The fact that the gaze is not directed accurately towards objects in the first days after birth, is due to an insufficient development of certain reflex connecting paths at the level of the cortex; the rapid development of precise movements of fixation, accommodation and convergence, is not compatible with empirical acquisition by trial and error.

The whole motor apparatus for ocular movement is essentially a reflex apparatus, controlled only with great difficulty by associative caprice, or by the will. We know how difficult it is to get a parafoveal fixation in the light or a foveal fixation in darkness, or to retain the fixation of the eye when a vivid and sudden excitation occurs in the periphery of the visual field, and how impossible it is to keep the eye at rest in darkness, even on a visible point, when this is single and faintly luminous.

Our knowledge of our ocular movements as such is very imperfect, and they can be controlled only by

[1] *Cf.* Henri Piéron, "L'orientation auditive latérale" (A critical survey and study of the theory of mechanism), *Année Psychologique*, XXIII, 1923, pp. 186-213.

[2] We may recall that the threshold of the impression of relief occurs with a separation (deviation of corresponding elements of two images) below the perceptible spatial differential threshold: a deviation below 3″ is enough to give a stereoscopic effect (*cf.* J. Coma Solà. "Les courants stellaires étudiés stereoscopiquement," *Scientia*, 1922, XVI, p. 217), while the most delicate spatial threshold corresponds to 30″ for two juxtaposed surfaces, and to 5″ for two lines end to end.

means of the reflex mechanisms that we succeed in arousing (parallelism of the ocular axes, for example, can be obtained by the representation of a distant object, or their convergence by the representation of an object close at hand).

We are consequently led to believe that, for sight even more than for hearing, spatial perception is the result of an awareness of ocular reflexes. It is the movement of the gaze up or down, to the right or the left, and accommodation or binocular convergence towards a relatively distant point, which furnish us with the corresponding ideas of direction and distance.

This conception finds solid support in the admirable studies of Gordon Holmes on patients with cerebral lesions, all of whom, in different degrees but in the same form, presented disturbances of visual orientation.[1]

In addition to some older cases, similar in every respect as regards symptomatology and with corresponding cerebral lesions (two patients of Inouye's wounded in the Russo-Japanese war, one of Riddoch's, in 1917, and several cases of vascular disease noted by Pick, Balint, and van Valkenburg), the seven cases of Holmes (one published with Smith and one with Horrax), two of which were followed by autopsy, furnish data which show remarkable agreement.[2]

In every case, after bilateral lesions of the cerebral hemispheres involving on both sides the area of the angular gyrus, similar disturbances appeared: there was an inability to judge whether one object was nearer or farther away than another; whether it was situated lower or higher, to the right or to the left. As a consequence, orientation in space was very much impaired, involving an incapacity to walk and avoid obstacles.

These disturbances, which were often accompanied

[1] Gordon Holmes, "Disturbances of Visual Orientation," *British Journal of Ophthalmology*, 1918, II, pp. 449-468 and pp. 506-516.

[2] I have given an outline of Gordon Holmes' observations in the *Journal de Psychologie*, 1921, XVIII, pp. 801-817.

by a derangement of visual attention, were not associated with an affection of sight itself, though in certain cases there was complete hemianopsia, hemianopsic scotomata or peripheral contractions, according to the nature and extent of the cerebral lesion. These disturbances were chance occurrences, since they were sometimes absent, and in numerous other cases where they existed there was generally no disturbance of the function of orientation.

But a disturbance of orientation was constantly accompanied by a disturbance of the ocular reflexes of fixation and convergence, of the reactions of accommodation and even of the reflex of blinking at the approach of an object.

The movements of the eyes were normal; they were even normally produced by excitation other than visual, for example under the influence of a noise, and especially under the influence of tactile or kinæsthetic excitation. Thus, when it was quite impossible for the patient to follow with his gaze the movement of a finger in front of him, he could generally follow his own finger very well, converging at its approach and even blinking at the sudden approach of his own hand; under the influence of visual excitation alone, the movements were inco-ordinated.

This apraxic disorder, which closely resembles the aphemic disturbances of verbal motor co-ordination, is regarded by Gordon Holmes as a consequence of the disturbance of the sense of visual orientation.

In my opinion, the terms must be reversed, and the disorder of orientation must be explained as a disturbance of the reflexes. As a matter of fact, the localization was possible when the reflexes were co-ordinated and adapted, for example under the influence of auditory, tactile or kinæsthetic stimuli. And the more pronounced disturbance—sometimes the only one presented—of the idea of distance coincided with a predominant disorder in the reflexes of binocular convergence.

The blind and persons affected with ocular paralysis succeed in orienting themselves in space without the reflexes of the eye, by means of other mechanisms. But when these ocular reflexes exist and are disturbed, they tend in their turn to disturb the idea of space, and to prevent correct orientation.

We can connect with these pathological data the fact that the normal mental representation of a direction implies an ocular attitude. It follows the adoption of this attitude and is impossible without it.[1]

Thus for sight as for hearing, for touch and for the labyrinthine function, the associative reactions of spatial perception, empirically acquired, are due to the awareness of spatial reflexes, innate reactions of localization. This does not mean that spatial perceptions cannot originate by the method of trial and error in the absence of these reflexes, and produce in their turn adapted localizing reactions. But the reflexes allow a much more rapid and precise acquisition. They at once give a significance to the local retinal sign and to binocular separation, whence the associative reaction of stereoscopy doubtless arises only through the medium of the motor reactions predetermined in the structure of the nerve tracts.[2]

Other and more complex forms of disorders of orientation may, however, appear, without disorders of the ocular reflexes—as when the praxic centres are deprived of the regulative data from the visual sphere. We have cited the study of Pierre Marie and Béhague on a syndrome of disorientation through deep frontal lesions. On the other hand, Mme Athanassio-Bénisty gives, as characteristics of parietal wounds, "disorders of the

[1] *Cf.* Grünbaum, "Représentations de la direction et mouvements des yeux," *Archives neerl. de Physiol.*, 1920, IV, 2 pp. 214-233.

[2] Relief was not studied in a sufficiently systematic fashion in the observations of Gordon Holmes, who asserts that stereoscopic vision is preserved, and depth perceived, when the patient cannot say which part of the visual field is in front and which behind. The impression of relief is hardly complete and satisfying when this is the case!

sense of orientation in space" (upper parietal and supra-marginal gyrus); the irregularity of these disorders in such lesions is certainly due to the fact that the symptom of disorientation is connected with an interruption of association paths of occipital origin, disturbing the usual spatial thought, and to a certain degree spatial conduct, if the data of visual origin which control the frontal praxic centres are insufficient or disordered. With the major functions which require the complex participation of numerous centres and paths, there are many points where a lesion may cause disturbances, though these may be more or less masked and relatively capable of compensation.

CHAPTER V

SOME FACTS RELATIVE TO THE NERVOUS MECHANISM OF THE INCITO-ASSOCIATIVE CONNECTIONS AND TO THE SWITCHING OF REACTIONS

To get an idea of the relations of the mental functions and the cerebral mechanism, we must make use of the elementary physiology of the nervous system. The morphological point of view led at first to errors and confusions which sufficiently explain the discredit attaching to the work of that pioneer of localization, Gall.

At one time, when the theory of neurones was systematically formulated, a number of writers thought that nothing would be easier than to explain all psychical processes in terms of physiology; sleeping and waking, attention and memory, association and the course of thought were all explained by the idea of amœboid movement, a movement of the cell extensions themselves, establishing or breaking the various connections, isolating the cells, or putting them in reciprocal communication. This, however, was merely to refer the whole mystery of mental activity to the cell elements by endowing them with a truly remarkable initiative.

But the intricacies of cell extensions did not long allow us to assign high explanatory value to seductive fantasies embroidered on the theme of amœbism. Even the neurone was compromised by the theory of neurofibrillar continuity, which explained the nervous system as a continuous network of interconnected threads sustained by the cell-bodies, like telegraph wires hung on posts, which nevertheless play a certain trophic part.

Whatever may be the case with the neurofibrils, which have been suspected of being an artificial phenomenon due to the methods of histological preparation, where a variety of chemical treatments involve colloidal precipitations, what we are certain of, physiologically, is the functional individuality of the neurones.

Thus, as Sherrington has shown, the periodicity of the impulses in an afferent nerve is not the same as that in the efferent nerve, along a reflex circuit; the centripetal excitation has not continued its progress along the centrifugal tract, but has aroused a response from a neurone, and this response has specific characteristics.

This specific character of responses is rendered more definite by a concept which we owe to the valuable work of Lapicque, that of 'chronaxy.'[1]

Chronaxy is a technical term for a duration of electrical excitation in a motor nerve or a muscle, such that the intensity of excitation necessary to reach the threshold of the response is twice as great as this liminal intensity (thence called 'rheobasic') with an indefinite duration of excitation. But the term acquires a general significance and value inasmuch as chronaxy is linked with the specific characters of the nervous impulse; it is a time constant representative of this impulse, which has a periodicity, a speed of transmission and a length of period, all variable. But the impulse should not be compared to a vibratory wave; it is a wave of electric disturbance transmitted along the nerve,[2] a wave

[1] For a survey, see L. Lapicque, "Principes pour une théorie du fonctionnement nerveux," *Revue générale des Sciences*, 1910, pp. 113-117.

[2] R. S. Lillie has given a physico-chemical example of a certain disturbance which was transmitted as a wave with a variable speed, like a nervous impulse. An iron wire placed in strong nitric acid, and then in a more dilute acid, is not attacked (this state is called 'passive'). When it is touched with a piece of iron an attack is produced at this point (activation),

of polarization, to follow Nernst's conception, which has been verified and rendered more definite by the labours of Lapicque, Cardot and Laugier.

But—and here is the important fact—the excitation of one element by another is related not only to the intensity of the electrical disturbance, but also to its own time constant. Lapicque has demonstrated, first, that each muscle has the same chronaxy as its nerve, and that if the chronaxy of one of the two was modified in any direction whatever, and all the more so if the two chronaxies were modified in opposite directions, the contraction of the muscle, under the influence of the excitation of the nerve, became more and more difficult to effect and for a certain relation between the chronaxies—when the one became double the other—could not be elicited at all (effect of curare); on the other hand a parallel variation of the two chronaxies did not change the excitability.

These relations of the nerve and the muscle suggest the relation of one neurone to another: the response of the neurone corresponding to the contraction of the muscular fibre is the production of an impulse; this response is the more easily aroused by an impulse coming from another neurone in proportion as the exciting impulse has a time constant closer to that of the excited neurone, and in proportion as these two neurones in connection are more perfectly 'isochronic,' in more exact 'syntony.'

Thus even with prolongations intricated in many connections, the excitation of a neurone will involve a selective response by predominant action on another neurone which is sufficiently isochronic: and so we get a reflex circuit. But if the exciting impulse reaches

with the usual active effervescence, which sweeps along the entire length of the wire (at a speed of 10 to 100 centimetres a second), and will be transmitted to another wire in contact with it, etc.; the passive state being re-established after the passage of the wave of activation (R. S. Lillie, "The Transmission of Physiological Influence in Nerve and Other Forms of Living Matter," *Scientia* 1920, No. 12, pp. 429-444).

great intensity, responses will be obtained in more and more heterochronic neurones, which corresponds to the laws of the irradiation and generalization of reflexes.

Except in the case of pathological actions, the chronaxies of the spinal neurones must remain quite fixed, so that the reactions have no great variability. But if the neurones can undergo more or less important modifications of their temporal constant, new isochronisms and heterochronisms will appear and the play of the syntonies will be modified; and thus the reactions may be completely changed.[1] But chronaxies vary with varying influences, not only those of toxic agents but also fatigue or physiological substances, such as adrenalin, etc. Moreover, a fundamental point, chronaxies vary under the influence of nervous action itself:[2] an ex-

[1] Thus Babinski's sign, which is characteristic of pyramidal lesions (and which consists in the substitution of an extension reflex of the toes in place of the flexion reflex normally elicited by excitation of the sole of the foot) is due, according to Bourguignon's observations, to a variation in chronaxy. The flexors of the toes have a chronaxy equal to that of the posterior tibial nerve, which ensures plantar sensibility, while the extensors have a chronaxy of half as much; thus it is normally the flexors which, being syntonized, respond to the plantar sensory excitation. But as a result of pyramidal lesions the chronaxy of the flexors diminishes while that of the extensors increases until its value is doubled. There is now an accord between the sensory nerve and the extensors, and the reflex response takes the form of extension (*cf.* G. Bourguignon, "La signification physiopathologique du signe de Babinski," *C. R. Ac. des Sciences*, July 20, 1925).

[2] Thus Mme Lapicque has proved that a modification of the chronaxy of a motor nerve under the influence of caffeine occurs only when the nerves are linked with the nervous centres, which must therefore be responsible for the modification of chronaxy (*C. R. Soc. de Biologie*, 1913, LXXIV, p. 32). More recently she has shown that the chronaxy of the peripheral motor nerves is doubled when the effects of chloroform or an encephalic re-section put the higher centres out of action; which demonstrates the influence of these centres on the value of the chronaxy ("Action des centres encéphaliques sur la chronaxie des nerfs périphériques," *C. R. Soc. de Biologie*, 1923, LXXXVIII, pp. 46-47).

Still more convincing is the observation of Bourguignon and Laugier which shows a reflex modification of chronaxy in man. Excitation of the extensor of the left index during arterial compression of the right arm produced an important modification of chronaxy ("Modification sexpérimentales de l'excitabilité par répercussion réflexe chez l'homme," *C. R. Soc. de Biologie*, 1923, LXXXVIII, pp. 265-270).

citation is capable not only of involving the proper response of the neurone, but also of contributing to a modification of the nature of this response by an action analogous to trophic action.

In particular, the excitation could have the effect of bringing together the characteristics of the impulse produced and those of the activating impulse, which would produce a greater facility, through repetition, for subsequent excitation—an attractive explanation of the well-known phenomenon of the facilitation of nerve tracts, or *Bahnung*, which is the basis of all the phenomena of habit and of memory.[1] The chronaxies of the higher neurones and of the cortical neurones—perhaps because they are subject to more numerous and more complex influences—appear to be the most variable.

We are dealing here with hypotheses which go beyond the facts but are in strict agreement with them, and which, since they are capable of verification by conceivable methods, are no longer mere speculations.

We may legitimately employ this method of explanation and, with Lapicque, relate the ideas of unequal and variable resistances of the 'synapses,' the points of juncture of the neurones, to the syntony of the nerve cells; the transmission at the level of the synapses symbolizes the excitation of the neurones by one another. The phenomena of 'facilitation'[2] and

[1] Delage has expressed this hypothesis as follows:—"When a neurone *a* has forced a neurone *b* to vibrate with it by reason of the intensity of the excitation and in spite of the difference between the vibratory mode of *b* and its own, it modifies in this way the mode of *b* and brings it nearer to its own. It causes this approximation for a considerable time, but *b* gradually recovers its original mode except for a slight remainder which continues to diminish slowly, without ever disappearing altogether ("Constitution des Idées," *Revue Philos.*, 1915, p. 299; reprinted as Chapter V, p. 111, in his book *Le Rêve*, Paris, 1920).

[2] 'Facilitation' which seems to be a mental effect of attention, has also a very exact physiological significance, shown in the study of cortical functions, by Graham Brown in particular. By stimulation of the motor point of the cortex, the excitability of neighbouring connected regions is augmented (but not if the association fibres are cut), which constitutes

those of inhibition may find their explanation in modifications of the nature of the impulse of a given neurone under the excito-modifying influence of other connected elements.

With the support of the physiologically established idea of the individuality of the neurones, and that of time constants allowing syntonized communications in a complex network (as we tend now to use the processes of wireless telegraphy 'with wires,' however paradoxical the expression may seem), we may examine, very rapidly, a few questions of sensory reception and of associativo-motor connection, in which both specificity of reception and switching of reactions must be involved.

A cold metallic point touches the skin; it gives rise to a sensation of contact, a sensation of cold and an impression concerning the location of the cutaneous region thus doubly excited. One nerve-ending has been affected, and thence proceeded the impulse conditioning the sensation of contact; another has also undergone a modification appearing as an impulse from which the sensation of cold arises. The two cells of the spinal ganglia, on which these peripheral nerve-endings depend, each enter into functional relation with a series of other relay neurones, to excite them in their turn and, finally, to stimulate in the ascending parietal convolution a specific incito-associative neurone of contact and one of cold, the specificity re-appearing at every level, by determined —and different—categories of reactions; but the same types of reaction will be released by all the elements of the afferent paths of the contact group and the cold group. Besides, each point touched gives rise to the excitation of a particular chain of neurones and this involves certain reactions having a different specificity,

'secondary facilitation,' just as for a certain time (ten seconds), the threshold of excitation is lowered by a brief preliminary excitation ("On the Phenomenon of Facilitation," *Quart. Journal of Exper. Physiol.*, 1915, IX, pp. 81-99, 117-130, 131-145; 1916, X, pp. 97-102, 103-143).

a local signature this time sensibly common to the two adjacent chains—because they are adjacent—and finishing at points which are very close together, of cold and of contact.

Vaso-motor and pilo-motor reflexes will characterize the cold excitation, as distinguished from the tactile excitation, and this in connection with the different groups of neurones excited by distinct spinal tracts, and having their own connections and isochronisms; bnt particular reflexes, scratching for example, may also be released by the two excitations, the muscular co-ordination being specifically modified according to the position of the nerve-endings excited at the surface of the skin, at every level of the chain of spinal encephalic neurones involved.[1]

The specificity of the retinal excitations with its translation into reflexes which are principally ocular and altogether different in type, constitutes a quite heterogeneous group, that of vision, in which the qualities of the sensations (brightness and colour) will also be accompanied by local signatures.

In every case, from the fact that a chain of neurones is set in operation, with all its own reaction processes, which depend on its connections and its chronaxic coefficient, there is a sensory specificity connected with the individuality of the responses. This represents the form that Müller's important principle of the specific energy of the nerves may take to-day.

Now, is there not a new quality which may arise, with a single chain of receptive neurones, from the fact of changes in the quantity of the excitation, the fact

[1] The local specificity—reactive in origin—is so distinct that at the time of the recovery of a severed peripheral nerve, when the fibres lose their way, as sometimes happens, and arrive in a cutaneous region different from that which they had formerly innervated. an excitation from this new region is referred to the old one; thus in the recovery of the sciatic nerve in a patient wounded in the war, the fibres innervating the heel and toes ended in the genital organs, and a contact undergone by those organs gave sensations localized in the foot (*cf.* André Thomas, "Restauration défecteuse des fibres sensitives, Topoparesthesies-synesthesies," *Revue Neurologique*, 1916, XX, III (1), pp. 305-311).

that the specific sensation presents different levels of intensity? Fechner's law has here taught us that these apparent increases in intensity occur less rapidly than those in the quantity of excitation: but this purely physiological law is characteristic, in a very general way, of the quantitative variation of an organic process produced by a given excitant; the process tends towards an impassable limit and its increase weakens progressively before approaching this limit. This roughly approximates to the logarithmic law, and the rate of increase of a negative variation, of a magnitude proportional to that of the nervous impulse to which it bears evidence, is in the form of an S curve (slow at first with acceleration and then weakening) as research on the excitation of the retina by light has shown.[1]

All along the receptive chain, as far as the cortical connecting neurones, the response—the sensation of which will be the associative interpretation, with its perceptive reactions—will thus increase as a function of the intensity of excitation according to a complex formula whose logarithmic law is almost represented by the graph of the middle range of the growth curve.[2] But how can these variations in the magnitude of the response be ascertained? Here the idea of quality makes its appearance.

We may suppose that a modification of reaction is due to a process of irradiation reaching reaction circuits

[1] Haas's researches (Leiden, 1903) cited by Victor Henri and Larguier des Bancels ("Sur l'interprétation de la loi de Weber-Fechner," *C. R. Soc. de Biologie*, 1912, LXXII, p. 1075, and *Archives de Psychologie*, 1912, XII, p. 329).

[2] At the same time the latent period of the reception diminishes according to a curve which some have tried to connect with a logarithm of Fechner's type, and which is really a kind of hyperbola. But this decrease results from a combination of complex phenomena, which, after having determined the general law, I am analysing for various sensations (*cf.* H. Piéron, "Recherches sur les lois de variation des temps de latence sensorielle en fonction des intensités excitatrices," *Année Psychologique*, 1914, XX, pp. 17-96; "Nouvelles recherches sur l'analyse du temps de latence sensorielle et sur la loi qui relie ce temps á l'intensité de l'excitation," *Idem*, 1922, XXII, pp. 58-132).

that are more and more heterochronic; each new extension being specific of one further degree of intensity of the sensation, whose increase is discontinuous by that very fact, the rise of one degree representing the value of a differential threshold. But the change in intensity often seems to be characterized not by an extension but by a modification of the reaction.[1] I have also suggested the hypothesis—which so far lacks any experimental support—that the augmentation of the intensity of response might be accompanied, in the cortical connecting neurones, by a progressive modification of the chronaxy changing the isochronisms (by a distant analogy with the movement of the length of the predominant wave in black-body radiation when the energy given out increases with the temperature). Thus a dog, which by the method of the conditioned reflex salivates for a sound of a certain pitch and intensity, can be trained not to salivate for a note of higher or lower pitch and also for the same note of higher or lower intensity, provided the difference reaches the value of the differential threshold, that is to say of the step corresponding to a modification in the nature of. the reaction circuits involved in the response — a step which would then represent the difference of chronaxy sufficient to pass from one of these circuits to another more perfectly isochronic.[2] Other hypotheses are possible. In any case, a different specificity of response must be implicated in order to add to the degrees of sensation connected with general and local qualities, the degrees connected with different intensities.

The practical value of these categories of qualities is

[1] When there is a judgment of identity or difference, it is because a particular associative reaction of the second order is occurring, conditioned by the primary reaction, whether the same or different; this is a gain in perceptive knowledge.

[2] *Cf.* H. Piéron, "Sur la signification physiologique des lois dites 'psychophysiques'" (Communication à la Société de Psychologie du 12 janvier 1922, *Journal de Psychologie*, 1922, XIX, pp. 365-370).

very unequal: the first inform us concerning the particular groups of stimuli (luminous, thermal, mechanical, vibratory and others), the second concerning the active intensity of the stimuli in operation. But our scale of intensities is composed of very unequal steps which are close together only for the middle of the scale, the most usual magnitudes of excitation (Weber's law of the constant proportional variation of the differential thresholds in comparison with absolute intensities of excitation being—very approximately—valid only for these middle values), and which are greatly increased at the upper and lower extremities.[1]

Furthermore, the appreciation of quantities of excitation can only become satisfactory when we have substituted local and more constant qualities for these intensive qualities of sensations, especially if well-chosen receptive areas are taken.

By making use of the capacity which discriminates two points seen by the fovea or, if need be, felt by the tips of the fingers, we render possible the reading of artificial scales in which we find a constant gradation serving as a common measure and movable at will from place to place. Scientific ingenuity has been able to submit to such scales almost all the phenomena that we were tempted to estimate according to the intensity of the sensation felt, with the sole exception of light, the idea of which is not yet freed from its

[1] Not only is the correspondence of degrees of reaction with the quantitative variations of excitation very imperfect, but there are also important modifications of organic origin even in the correspondence of the magnitude of the afferent physiological process with that of the process of stimulation; and this holds true at variable levels of the chain of receptive neurones (under vascular influences, for example) but especially in the incito-associative connection area of the cortex. Here the phenomena of facilitation and inhibition (which appear as variations of attention) play a large part. In sleep, when the affective area does not intervene to reinforce the selective sensations, the inhibition of the connecting function is almost complete. Very intense sensations succeed in filtering into the associative region only like a ray of light under a door, scarcely influencing the filiform course of the thought of the dream.

primitive sensory envelope.[1] Measurement originates from the qualitative distinction of juxtaposed chains of receptive elements to a specific response, to which the discontinuity of number is adapted, the other qualities[2] (the pitch of sounds, the chromatic shade of lights, etc.) being also utilized, but rarely in methods of approximation. It is, in a general way, conditioned by the number of incito-associative receptive neurones, selectively excitable, having specific connections and able to produce distinct motor, verbal, evocative and other reactions.

Since a differentiation is biologically possible only through the passage from one reaction to another, discontinuity is an inevitable law; when we are confronted by continuous phenomena, perception is effected step-wise in space and time. Whatever may be the appearance of subjective continuity connected with a passive attitude, psychological phenomena are essentially discrete; or, if it is preferred, our psychological knowledge of phenomena is fundamentally discontinuous—a fact which is related to the mechanisms concerned.

[1] It is not generally realized that light is not a physical phenomenon but the psycho-physiological effect of certain kinds of radiation, and that thus the idea of luminous intensity shares in all the uncertainties of the intensive qualities of the sensations (*cf.* H. Piéron, "La photométrie est-elle possible?" *Revue de Mois*, 1919, 116, pp. 208-215, "Des principes physiologiques qui doivent présider à toute étude de la lumiére," *Revue générale des Sciences*, October 15 and 30, 1920).

[2] These qualities are also conditioned by a selective excitation of specific neurones with their own associative and reactive connections, the number of perceptible shades or musical notes is limited by the number of the connecting neurones separately excitable by a variation in the frequency of light rays or sound vibrations.

Part III

THE VERBAL FUNCTION AND THOUGHT

(The Cerebral Mechanism of Language and Aphasia)

INTRODUCTION

It is when we try to represent the cerebral functioning of language and symbolic thought that we put our general conceptions of psycho-physiology and of cerebrology to the most severe test.

Theories are numerous and are the subject of violent controversy, and as a result of over-simple schematization many people have become hopelessly confused.

But from the various efforts which have been made and the immense stock of observations accumulated on the disorders of language, and on aphasia, it is possible to disentangle some essential data, which may serve as a guide; and if we look at the question in the light of the modern dynamic view, whether physiological or psychological, the confusion may be dissipated, and old views which we are too often content to reject without seeing that they express, though in an inadequate form, incontestable facts, will be interpreted in a different sense.

Without entering in detail into their history, we may recall the three great stages of the evolution of theories of aphasia.[1]

In 1861, Broca gave a masterly description of the disorder which he called aphemia, and which consists

[1] The important summary of the matter in François Moutier's thesis (*L'Aphasie de Broca*, 1908) may be profitably consulted.

in the abolition of articulated language with preservation of the activity of articulation and of the "general faculty of language," and he indicated as the seat of the correlative lesion the foot of the third left frontal. In 1869, Bastian described verbal deafness, a disturbance of the auditory comprehension of language without injury to audition. Wernicke indicated, in the first left temporal, the centre whose lesion involved the loss of 'auditory images' of words. Then verbal blindness and agraphia were isolated; the types of aphasia increased and explanatory diagrams were sketched. With his admirable lucidity Charcot elaborated a doctrine which became classic, and outlined a general diagram on which numbers of others were modelled.

Dejerine, who adopted the general views of Wernicke, denied the localization of writing, only admitting the existence of the centres which seemed to him innate. Yet he located the visual images of words in the angular gyrus. And he distinguished aphasias in which inner language is affected, through destruction of the centres where the images of words are stored, from those in which, owing to sub-cortical lesions,[1] there is a simple isolation of the centres, causing a pure aphemia, a pure verbal deafness and a pure verbal blindness.

Finally, in 1906, Pierre Marie entered the field and endeavoured to combat the distortion of facts with a constructive theory. He showed that aphasia of the Broca type was a total aphasia, and maintained that the foot of the third frontal played no part in the function of language. For him 'Broca's aphasia' covers an incapacity for verbal articulation, an 'anarthria' conditioned by a lesion located somewhere in a very large quadrilateral including the insula and the lenticular area, and a true aphasia, an intellectual disorder of the

[1] Dejerine was obliged, however, to recognize that the sub-cortical lesions did not signify aphasia with no disturbance of the internal language: pure aphasias were accompanied by widespread cortical lesions (Pitres, Ladame) and disorders of the internal language were noted in cases where there was no cortical lesions whatever.

comprehension and use of language, connected with a temporo-parietal lesion, in 'Wernicke's zone.' There are no verbal images, or motor images any more than

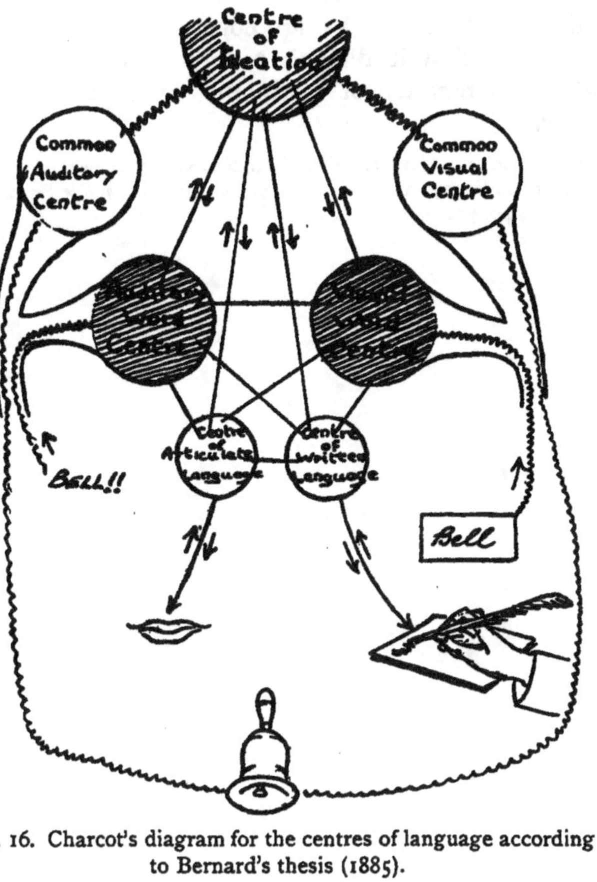

FIG. 16. Charcot's diagram for the centres of language according to Bernard's thesis (1885).

there are auditory or visual images; hence there is no aphemia, verbal deafness or verbal blindness.[1]

At present, in an atmosphere of thought impregnated with Bergson's powerful critique, so quickly assimilated that it has become impersonal, it is the intellectual

[1] Since the experience of the War, the reality of the classic verbal blindness has been recognized by Pierre Marie and his pupils.

analysis of the function of language, such as that attempted by Head, which has come to the front; and we are returning to the profound views of Hughlings Jackson,[1] which were obscured by the brilliance and prestige of Charcot. We are concerned with the facts, but we still find it difficult to break away from the bonds of sympathy or antipathy in regard to the theories.

[1] See the studies of Head and that of R. Mourgue ("La méthode d'étude des affections du langage d'après Hughlings Jackson," *Journal de Psychologie*, 1921, XVIII, pp. 752-764).

CHAPTER I

THE ACTUAL DATA CONCERNING APHASIA

LET us consider, first of all, the nature of the facts revealed by pathology.

Are there verbal blindnesses, verbal deafnesses, aphemias and agraphias? What is the effect of these disorders on thought? How are they inter-related? Can they exist in a pure state, either at the outset or as the result of a general disturbance? These are questions which must be considered without prejudice and without theoretical controversy, before we discuss the problem of mechanisms or the points in which current notions require correction. We will therefore examine the facts first from the point of view of the four forms of aphasia distinguished in Charcot's theory, and then from that of complex aphasias, in their relation to thought.[1]

1. *Verbal Blindness*

Numerous observations establish beyond doubt the existence of an isolated disorder bearing on the verbal comprehension of graphic signs.

In one case, which we have elsewhere described, the incapacity to understand and to read words occurred from the very start, accompanied by a right hemianopsia.

[1] We shall have occasion, in what follows, to allude to personal observations on cases of injury or illness in the course of the War. These observations were published in a study ("La notion des centres co-ordinateurs cérébraux et le mécanisme du langage") which appeared in the *Revue Philosophique* (1921, 46th year; *cf.* pp. 106-123).

As the hemianopsia did not affect the macula,[1] there was no visual disorder. Objects were well recognized, and so were designs, as well as most of the letters and even some words. Little by little, by regression, oral reading developed, as did the capacity of interpreting in movements of articulation the images corresponding to the phonemes, comprehension following the enunciation of the words; the graphic copy—even with different signs—had always been sufficiently well preserved (transcription of the printed text).

The greatest disturbance was in the synthetic comprehension of phrases, it was less for words, and least of all for letters; there was a slighter difficulty in oral reading, and a minimal difficulty in graphic transcription. At the same time it was a man with a musical education—there was a total lack of comprehension of the nature of the notes in the key of F, and a partial lack of comprehension of the notes in the key of G.

Here was a case of blindness, not absolutely complete but very marked, not accompanied by agraphia, aphemia, or word-deafness, or by disorders of the intelligence. The patient understood and wrote—without being able to read his work again—several languages; he wrote spontaneously or to dictation, at least with his right hand, though not with his left.

This observation was in every way paralleled by a certain number of others which have been published since the first account by Dejerine[2] in 1892. Dejerine's clinical description of this syndrome is scrupulously exact.

The comprehension of numbers and symbols (R. F., for example, cards, dominoes, flags, etc.) is preserved, sometimes with a lack of comprehension affecting all

[1] There are pseudo-alexias through loss of macular vision, through a considerable diminution of visual acuity: very large letters are recognized, while small print gives a confused vision.

[2] *Cf.* particularly the case, where the patient afterwards recovered, cited by Dejerine in *Séméiologie des affections du système nerveux*, 1914, note on p. 94.

the letters (literal blindness);[1] the name of the patient is generally recognized, but not always. There can be complete incapacity to pronounce the syllables and the words seen. Finally the transcription of a printed text may itself be affected.

Cases have been mentioned where verbal blindness was accompanied by an inability to name the objects seen[2]—although they were recognized. Cases of this type often involve more complex disorders, such as that of naming objects felt, and then real recognition is doubtful: it might be a matter of asymbolia or general agnosia. But sometimes it certainly seems that the incapacity to name the words seen constitutes an isolated disturbance, since the objects are recognized; a functional associative disturbance would prevent their being called by name, the attention being fixed on their evocation by means of sight.[3]

We may note, that right hemianopsia due to lesion

[1] In this connection, there are cases in which literate individuals can read the word as a whole by oral repetition and sometimes understand it, without being able to separate it into syllables and recognize the letters separately (*cf.* J. Froment and A. Devic, "Contribution à l'étude de la cécité, de la surdité verbale et de la paraphasie," *Bull. et Mém, de la Soc. méd. des Hôpit. de Paris*, May 22, 1913, Vol. II, pp. 1010-1017).

[2] *Cf.* Von Rosenfeld, "Zur optisch-sensorischen Aphasie," *Neur. Centr.*, May 1, 1901, p. 395. Optical aphasia was described by Freud in 1904.

[3] In a case of a bullet-wound in the left hemisphere, with trephining at the level of the angular gyrus near the exit (with a frontal entrance), a homonymous hemianopsia was accompanied by "visual agnosia characterized by the recognition of objects with inability to name them"; without verbal blindness, words read being understood (P. Jeandelize, "Une forme d'aphasie visuelle," *Rev. méd. de l'Est*, 1920, p. 325). But, in general, optical aphasia is accompanied by verbal blindness. Very clear cases have recently been described by Louis Poussep and by Crouzon and Valence. In the first, followed by autopsy (which revealed a softening of the angular gyrus and of the superior occipital convolution) objects were named as soon as they were touched but could not be named when they were only seen; in the second, a clear verbal blindness persisted during the retrocession of optical aphasia (difficulty in getting the names of objects and colours without error, in spite of correct recognition), and a curious loss of the power of, as it were, "reading objects" (*cf.* L. Poussep, "Contribution aux recherches sur la localisation de l'aphasie visuelle," *Presse* médicale, 1923, pp. 564-565;—Crouzon and Valence, "Un cas d'alexie pure," *Bull. et Mém. de la Soc. Médicale des Hôpitaux*, 1923, pp. 1145-1149).

of the optic radiations of the left hemisphere almost constantly coexists with verbal blindness.[1] This is an interesting fact in connection with the localization of the lesions, and we shall return to it when we come to deal with the problem of verbal localization. In one of my cases, however, which was not due to the usual pathogeny, as a result of small lesions due to shock, I found verbal blindness without hemianopsia.

There are, therefore, verbal blindnesses which are incontestably pure, with differences in the extent of the disturbance. They do not exist only in theory, but a clinical reality.[2]

2. *Verbal Deafness*

Though pure verbal blindness is well-established, we cannot say the same of pure verbal deafness, though a lack of comprehension of language is common among aphasic patients.

Dejerine, in 1914, had difficulty in collecting eight cases of pure verbal deafness without peripheral disturbance of the auditory apparatus. But since in certain of these cases there was a bilateral lesion of the temporal lobes, with a central impairment of hearing, it may be suggested that the lack of verbal comprehension was due to insufficiently distinct audition or confused reception.

In 1898, however, Liepmann reported a case of pure verbal deafness which had lasted fourteen months and in which the autopsy revealed only a recent hæmorrhagic centre, the cause of death—masking a more ancient lesion—in the white matter of the left temporal lobe, with no injury to the right temperal lobe. Audition

[1] In a left-handed individual, however, pure verbal blindness was accompanied by left homonymous hemianopsia, indicating a lesion of the right hemisphere (*cf.* J. Bollack and L. Hartmann, *Société d'Ophthalmologie*, January 15, 1921).

[2] "Pure verbal blindness, or more accurately, pure alexia, exists," says Chatelin (*Les blessures du cerveau*, 2nd edit., 1918, p. 109).

was not affected, as in one of the cases of Hérard and Maillard (1910), where there was no autopsy.

But though from a clinical point of view we may neglect pure verbal deafness, which is very rare, its mere existence, even as an exception, loses none of its value from the theoretical point of view.[1]

In these cases there is correct speech, complete preservation of spontaneous writing, and normal comprehension of written texts with oral reading unaffected. But speech cannot be repeated and writing to dictation is impossible. Articulation by the phonemes heard is lacking, as well as graphic translation, and, at the maximum, there is no comprehension of phrases and words.

But nearly always—and hence is derived Wernicke's and Dejerine's idea of sensory aphasia—when the words pronounced are not understood, the words read are not any better understood. This common syndrome has been conceived, on the lines of Charcot's theory, as a combination of verbal blindness with verbal deafness. This is questionable, as we shall see; but it must be noted that both are susceptible of degree. We have indicated the variability of failure in visual comprehension. From the auditory point of view, the name of the patient can be recognized, sometimes also his Christian name, sometimes a few words. There may be a lack of comprehension of foreign languages only; there may be a lack of comprehension limited to certain words or to complex phrases. Usually there are several words which are understood and which cause the rest to be guessed at, naturally with errors; grammatical subtleties, conjugation and syntax, escape the patient.

Generally comprehension is more affected than the

[1] Another of Pierre Marie's pupils, Ch. Foix, in a discussion at the Société de Neurologie de Paris, reported that he had found a case of pure verbal deafness, as a relict of a more complete auditory agnosia (*Revue Neurologie*, 1924, XXXI (ii), p. 500).

repetition of words or writing to dictation. But it can happen that repetition is electively affected, more than comprehension. A very good example of this came under our observation and its interpretation deserves to be discussed.

When there is no coexisting aphemia, there may indeed be speech, sometimes correct (pure verbal deafness, slight disturbances) and sometimes—in the ordinary case—with paraphasia (one word being said for another) or jargonophasia (completely unintelligible phrases).

The variations noticed between one case and another may also occur in the history of a single case, either through progressive amelioration or through aggravations (series of ictuses). In fact, certain forms are regarded as possible only by way of residue.

But whatever its origin, which is very important clinically, for theoretical purposes the occurrence of a dissociation on any occasion makes it imperative that we should not neglect it. And it is an incontestable fact that though verbal deafness is not usually found in the pure state, its intensity may vary independently in relation to other allied disturbances, not only phonic or graphic, but even in relation to those of verbal blindness.

If in weakened forms we always found more verbal blindness than deafness, and if the order of disappearance or of reappearance were always the same, we might suppose that they were various degrees of one injury. But this is not so. In some cases auditory comprehension or the repetition of speech appears to predominate; in others reading aloud, a more vulnerable activity, whose development, moreover, is often very slight; and finally, in others, and these are the most frequent, with visual comprehension; this indicates that the two processes are possibly independent, in spite of their clinical conjunction, quite apart from the question as to whether, in certain cases, the double injury may or may not arise from the same mechanism.[1] This dissociation scarcely allows us to assume the existence of a single type of aphasia, varying only in degree. It might be a matter of a complex with unequal participation of the components. We must say then that verbal deafness is a disturbance which, clinically, is found only exceptionally in the pure state, but which may constitute a relatively independent element of a complex clinical syndrome.

3. *Aphemia*

Though verbal blindness is not very frequent in the pure state and verbal deafness is extremely rare, aphemia—in the sense given it by Broca, though his principal case did not conform to the definition—Dejerine's sub-cortical motor aphasia, Pierre Marie's anarthria, constitutes a frequent disturbance of language, either primary, or as a relic of a more complex aphasia.

In aphemia, language is understood, mental reading is perfect, and mimicry and writing supplement the incapacity for oral expression. The words which the patient wants to pronounce are known: and if he is a person of sufficient education, he can even indicate the number of syllables or of letters of the word which he cannot enunciate.

Aphemia is sometimes associated with agraphia, the incapacity to write words, which are, however, known graphically and understood when read. But as aphemia is generally accompanied by right hemiplegia, cursive writing cannot be followed; we may note, then, in most cases that the left hand succeeds in tracing awkwardly the responses which are impossible orally. More often

[1] In Moutier's Case No. 33, for example (p. 692), we note that the execution of written orders, even when complicated, was always perfectly correct, whereas there were errors in the execution of the same orders when indicated orally. The reverse is the ordinary rule. In one of my own cases repetition was more difficult than reading aloud, and this is not exceptional.

the aphemia is associated with verbal deafness and blindness, and is then complicated by complete agraphia. In the weakened forms, some words can be pronounced, but the construction of phrases, syntax and conjugations are impossible.

There are aphemias with loss of those elements of internal language that Dejerine regards as the motor images of verbal articulation, distinct from pure aphemias with preservation of these elements. The former involve a disturbance of comprehension in reading, a slight disturbance in audition, an inability to write spontaneously or to take dictation, though the power to copy printed matter remains unimpaired, and an inability to indicate the number of syllables in a word (Proust-Lichtheim test). The last incapacity is the important fact, indicating loss of images of articulation. But it should be noted that as long as the auditory evocation of words is preserved, the number of syllables can still be indicated, and the number of letters in the case of visual evocation.[1] On the other hand, when we find disturbances of audition or of verbal vision, we can scarcely talk of aphemia alone. The criticism of aphemia of Pierre Marie, who treats these cases merely as relatively weakened complex aphasias, with a predominance of the disturbance of speech which he calls anarthria, is evidently justified.

There are pure aphemias or aphemias associated with other disorders of language. There are no grounds for differentiating pure aphemias with or without loss of 'motor images.' These are theoretical conceptions—with an anatomical representation which has been recognized as erroneous by Dejerine himself—which became mixed up with the facts and distorted them. Pierre Marie has enabled us to remove a dangerous source of confusion.

[1] *Cf.* J. Froment and O. Monod, "L'épreuve de Proust-Lichtheim-Dejerine," *Revue de Médécine*, 1913, XXXIII, pp. 280-295.

4. *Agraphia*

Dejerine, following Wernicke, holds that there are disturbances of writing among aphasic patients, but not agraphia as an independent syndrome; and this for theoretical reasons, since he objects to the identification of the mechanisms of speech and writing.[1]

These disorders, he contends, arise either from a disturbance of internal language among motor aphasics or from a sensory aphasia; writing is preserved in the 'pure' syndromes, *pure* verbal deafness (except, of course, in dictation) *pure* verbal blindness and *pure* aphemia only.

Writing, on this view, is also always affected, whatever the manner of writing, with the left hand or with the right, and, among motor aphasics who have lost their internal language, agraphia would develop parallel to aphemia, and disappear with it.

But these assertions are not borne out by the facts: in one of my own cases I found aphemia without aphasia of comprehension, accompanied by agraphia; and the agraphia was still very marked when the aphemia had almost completely vanished. There was, then, no parallelism, and the two forms of verbal motor expression occurred independently.

On the other hand, in a case of pure verbal blindness, cursive writing was perfectly preserved, but the patient did not know how to write with his left hand, for he had never practised writing with this hand, and endeavoured

[1] At first Dejerine assumed the existence of a cortical verbal blindness, with destruction of the visual images of words without verbal deafness and characterized by agraphia, which accompanied this form of verbal blindness (*cf.* J. Dejerine, "Contribution à l'étude anatomo-pathologique et clinique des différentes variétés de cécité verbale," *Mémoires de la Société de Biologie*, 1892, pp. 62-90).—Dejerine et André Thomas, "Sur un cas de cécité verbale avec agraphie suivi d'autopsie," *Revue neurologique*, July 15, 1904, pp. 655-664). Later, he connected agraphia with the sensory aphasia of Wernicke, a combination of cortical verbal blindness and deafness (Dejerine, "L'agraphie," *Progrès Médical*, July 13, 1912, p. 344).

to draw graphic symbols where visual evocation failed him.[1]

Thus the agraphia of the right and left hands is clearly not parallel. Moreover Pitres records a case of agraphia of the right hand without paralysis, with the power of writing with the left hand, a pure motor agraphia during a regression of aphemia;[2] and other analogous cases have been observed.[3] Though such cases are rare, the fact that they exist is enough to establish the existence of an autonomous mechanism. This is a point on which we insisted in connection with verbal deafness, in opposition to Pierre Marie's negative view and in favour of Dejerine's theory. Against Dejerine's denial based on one of Wernicke's theories, we can only repeat it again.

Pure agraphia—in so far as it is a verbal syndrome—may also accompany apraxic disorders without paralysis, the inability to perform habitual complex movements, as in the case of a left-handed patient who had learned to write with the right hand and with whom a left hemiplegia was accompanied by apraxia and agraphia.[4]

Naturally there are degrees in agraphia as in aphemia; letters and numbers can be written, but not words, and still less phrases. The name, the year, the place and the date of birth are often retained.

In general, spontaneous writing and writing to dictation evolve on parallel lines, but copying even printed texts transcribed in cursive hand is always better, be-

[1] In certain cases of pure verbal blindness, writing can be done with the left hand, as in the case of a right hemiplegia observed by Pélissier and Salès (*Revue neurologique*, 1913, XXI, II, p. 118), with a general tendency to reversal, by reproducing the graphic mechanisms of the right hand, which are imagined and transferred to the symmetrical hand.

[2] *Cf.* A. Pitres, "Consideration sur l'agraphie à propos d'une observation nouvelle d'agraphie motrice pure," *Revue de Médecine*, 1884, pp. 855-873 and *Congrès de Lyon*, 1894.

[3] *Cf.* Van Gehuchten and Van Gorp, *Bulletin de l'Academie de Médecine de Belgique*, March, 1914.

[4] *Cf.* F. Seiler, "Über einen Fall von reiner Agraphie bei einem an linksseitiger Hemipareseleidenden Linkshänder," *Korrespondenzblätter f. Schweizer Aerzte*, 1913, XLVII, pp. 1541-1558.

cause there is something more mechanical about it, as Dejerine remarks. In the most serious cases, the copying is done like a drawing, and printed letters are slavishly reproduced.

In the lightest forms, only certain failings are observed.[1]

Agraphia, which exists in complex aphasias, may be the only disorder accompanying verbal blindness.

Indeed, it seems that the existence of agraphia in cases affected with pure verbal blindness is connected with insufficiency of instruction or of graphic practice. Writing has not become automatic with them; it remains a drawing, a copy of a model visually evoked. When this evocation fails, writing cannot be performed; and then patients are very anxious to be given a model, and if necessary will fetch one, when they come across a letter they can no longer write.

This happened in a case of shell-shock which came under my observation. In literate persons, on the other hand, verbal blindness does not in the least disturb automatic writing of the right hand, but it may disturb attempts at writing with the left hand.

5. *The Aphasic Complexes and the Intellectual State*

We find isolated disturbances of visual or auditory comprehension, of oral or graphic expression, but usually there is a complex disturbance with a variable predominating factor; sometimes the aphasia is total and complete. When we are dealing with well delimited agraphic disturbances or verbal blindness, the reverberation of these on behaviour may be relatively negligible; especially, of course, if the patient has had only a rudimentary education. But even in aphemia, even in pure verbal deafness, it seems, according to the very

[1] An inability to write the name of objects seen has even been recorded as an isolated disorder analogous to an inability to pronounce the name of objects thus perceived (*cf.* Sciamanna, *R. Ac. di Med. di Roma*, April 28, 1901).

rare records available on this point, the disturbance of communication may be reduced by the use of writing, and speech would appear not to be affected at all.

When the disturbance is more extensive, this seems no longer to hold good. Though there is nothing in the fact to justify Dejerine's distinction between injuries of comprehension or of expression with loss of internal language and those without such loss—the distinction only holds between entirely isolated disturbances of a single function, and more or less extended disturbances in a complex whole—are there any intellectual disturbances in aphasias of the ordinary type which for Pierre Marie would be the true aphasias even without aphemia? Do we find any evidence that what is impaired is a higher function of the comprehension of language?

Evidently cases exist in which comprehension and expression are deeply affected, though the mechanisms of sensory reception or motor expression are not touched. These are cases of insanity, and here we find reactions with no relation to what is said to the patient, incoherent talk, and incomprehensible jargonophasia.

But aphasia is not insanity, a point on which Pierre Marie and his pupil Moutier strongly insist. Though they admit the existence of general intellectual disorders among aphasic patients—disorders of attention, memory, will etc.—they recognize that it is the intellectual function of language which is solely or at least principally affected.

With regard to general disorders—in cases of arteriosclerosis with cerebral thrombosis or hæmorrhage, or in cases of traumata and cerebral lesions—there is no cause for surprise. There is of necessity a general disturbance of cerebral functioning in these organic cases; of this there can be no question.

With regard to verbal intelligence, where comprehension of language is impaired, we may say that the intelligence is disordered if the function of 'comprehension' is affected *as such:* but if the behaviour shows correct adaptation to circumstances, to new conditions, when these, the object of sensory knowledge, require the evocation of sentiments, attitudes, and acts, without necessarily involving verbal signs, we are concerned only with a disorder of comprehension which is purely verbal. Indeed, there are many facts which establish the persistence of intelligent behaviour among aphasic patients.

We can call verbal comprehension 'intelligence'; this is a matter of definition. It is useless to argue here about terminological conventions. But, in reality, setting aside the word 'intelligence,' we are faced by the assertion that language is a single function disturbed in a single way. Now facts have shown that language involves various functions, the primitive functions of auditory comprehension and oral expression, and the functions, acquired later and not universal, of comprehension of the graphic signs of writing. And in each of these functions, we see that the loss or return operates according to the general law stated by Ribot: the new is more vulnerable than the old, and the complex than the simple.[1]

A slight disorder of reading will be shown in a failure to understand phrases whose sense is governed by the position of the words or by a conjugation of the verb; a deeper disturbance will efface the comprehension of words which are unusual and abstract; the patient's name will remain understood the longest. Sometimes the recognition of letters will be effaced before that of the last words and sometimes it will persist longest,

[1] This is a fact which has often been remarked, and we have come across several examples of it. The fact of comprehending only a few words in a phrase and guessing wrongly results from a verbal deficit and not from a generalized intellectual weakening, as Henri Dufour correctly observes. "These patients," he says, "are exactly in the position of a normal individual to whom a text is read in the following way: 'We . . . on the other hand, and . . . common . . . all categories . . . that,' etc. The missing words make the text incomprehensible, and there is no necessity to appeal to an intellectual deficit" (*cf.* "Hémiplégie cérébrale gauche avec aphasie," *Revue neurologique*, 1910, II, pp. 657-660).

which may be connected with the methods used in the learning of reading or the degree of intelligence or automatism in reading. But this whole hierarchy of disorders in reading may coincide with a perfect comprehension of the subtleties of spoken language.

If there were only one way of understanding language, such a dissociation would be impossible; but its existence seems undeniable.

In the same way, the return of speech may occur through the use of infinitives and substantives, in a telegraphic style or in pidgin English, while there will be normal comprehension of phrases read or understood in their grammatical complexity.

It is none the less true that the usual cases of aphasia, especially clear when they are not complicated with aphemia, or with a disorder of verbal expression, Pierre Marie's true aphasias or Wernicke's aphasias, involve a deep disturbance of the verbal function as a whole, comprehension and thought. Speech, correct from the point of view of elocution, is an incomprehensible rigmarole, to such a degree that patients may be treated as insane and confined—which would not occur if they were aphemic. Any thought requiring the use of signs and symbols is impossible.

There is a disturbance of internal language in sensory aphasias, says Dejerine, through loss of images; there is an intellectual disorder, an injury to verbal thought, independently of any image, says Pierre Marie. This is a question of interpretation, a problem of the mechanisms employed, and a matter which we shall have to examine.

CHAPTER II

THE PSYCHO-PHYSIOLOGICAL MECHANISMS OF LANGUAGE AND VERBAL THOUGHT

WE are confronted by two kinds of functions, those of motor expression and those of sensory comprehension, and we must consider how we ought to envisage the mechanism of these functions, which has been the object of such lively controversy and of such profound disagreement. We shall thus have to test the value of the idea of verbal images, rejected by Pierre Marie, motor images, and auditory or visual images, and to discover whether it is not necessary to give these expressions a sense different from the usual one—supposing they have a sense—or to substitute for them more comprehensive ideas. Finally we shall see how the connection between thought and language may be conceived, how we should envisage the nature of internal language and its rôle in mental functioning as a whole, and how aphasia of the current type, that of Wernicke, in its sensory and intellectual setting, can be interpreted.

1. *The Confusion involved in the Motor Image, and the Idea of Motor Co-ordination Centres*

The Apraxias

Broca regarded aphemia as the consequence of a lesion of the convolution of language, where he located this faculty. Wernicke introduced the idea of localized verbal motor images in the posterior part of the third left frontal. With Charcot and Ballet this idea became classic, aphemia being defined as the impossibility of evoking the motor images of articulation.

What then do these authors mean by a motor image? An auditory or visual image is a mnemonic representation of impressions of sound or light which constitute perception; the auditory and visual images of the words are localized in autonomous centres which are connected with the external world only by a single line in a centripetal direction: these are only centres of impression. But Broca's convolution and the foot of the second frontal, which are the centres of speech and writing, are motor centres, centres of expression, connected with the external world by a centrifugal line, and they are also centres of impression in part and hence connected with the external world by a second, centripetal line. In Charcot's diagram, the centre of articulate language is connected by this double line with the mouth which pronounces the word (see fig. 16, p. 151).

The seat of the images of articulation thus appears under a double aspect, motor and sensory, without any indication, as for hearing and sight, of an intermediate receptive stage between the periphery and the verbal centre (the common visual centre anterior to the visual centre of words, and the common auditory centre preceding the auditory centre of words).

We have here a singularly confused conception and the confusion has never been properly cleared up. 'Motor images' of words are freely rejected or assumed, although the term conceals two different meanings, the motor and the sensory. Dejerine, who distinguishes aphemias according as they are accompanied or not by the loss of motor images of articulation, which, with the auditory images (in the first instance) and the visual images (of decidedly secondary importance) constitute the idea of the word used in internal language, does not specify the nature of these images, which he localizes in Broca's centre. He declares that when we think with our auditory images, "at the same time as we hear the words resounding clearly in our inner consciousness, we are more or less conscious of the movements necessary for pronouncing them, the auditory image awakening the corresponding motor image." Universalizing, like Egger, his own type of inner speech, he refuses to admit that one or other may predominate as was implied, and he asserts that "we all think in the same way." "Think anything concrete," he adds, "and immediately we hear the words resound in our ears, at the same time as we have the idea of the necessary movements for pronouncing them."[1]

This view is entirely rejected by Pierre Marie, whose pupil Moutier expresses himself thus: "The image, then, is a succession of movements that we imagine, that we feel prepared to realize and do realize. It is the knowledge of the movement required to utter this word, the outline of this movement and this movement itself. In reality, we have no presentiment of the movements necessary for the articulation of a word. Let us ask ourselves: are we conscious of the position it is absolutely necessary to give to the glottis, the tongue, the cheeks, and the lips to pronounce a given word? Do we know how to *will* this position? Have we even the vaguest and remotest idea of what the mechanism of this verbal and vocal elaboration is? No."[2] And in the same way Froment and Monod declare that introspection does not in any way reveal the existence of verbo-motor images; according to them we cannot imagine the movements that we are going to effect; there are only unconscious motor habits.[3]

This general denial on the part of Moutier, and of Froment and Monod, really involves two distinct affirmations: 1, there are no images of verbal articula-

[1] *Séméiologie des affections du système nerveux*, pp. 115-116.

[2] *L'aphasia de Broca*, p. 243.

[3] J. Froment and O. Monod, "Du langage articulé chez l'homme normal et chez l'aphasique," *Archives de Psychologie*, 1913, No. 46, pp. 1-20.

tion; 2, language operates without the intervention of images of articulation. With regard to the first point, the negation based on personal introspection is obviously without value. Numerous objective data, the result of many experiments in controlled introspection,[1] justify the conclusion that in general there are kinæsthetic representations as there are auditory or visual ones, and that there are in particular kinæsthetic representation for the movements of verbal articulation.

It has been supposed that only kinæsthetic sensations exist, not mnemonic evocations of these sensations, that is to say, representations or images: thus to imagine a movement would be to accomplish it, or at least to outline it, and, in fact, when we imagine a movement, it is rare for the muscles involved in this movement to remain in repose. But, on the one hand, there is a discrepancy between the extent of an imagined movement, which may be extremely variable, and the real movement, if there is a movement; on the other hand, the illusion of those who have had limbs amputated clearly shows the possibility of motor representations without movement.

Now kinæsthetic representations of articulation behave exactly like all other kinæsthetic representations; they may become hallucinatory in the dream and in certain forms of delirium, and generally we are able to imagine the articulation of one phoneme while actually pronouncing a totally different one.[2] But the capacity for kinæsthetic representation varies

[1] Claparède, in defending the reality of motor images and verbo-motor images, very justly recalls the researches of Segal, G. E. Müller, and Koffka among others (Ed. Claparède, "Existe-t-il des images verbo-motrices?", *Archives de Psychologie*, 1913, No. 49, pp. 93-103). We may also refer to the results of G. Saint-Paul's fruitful enquiries, *Le langage intérieur et les paraphasies*, Paris, 1904.

[2] Thus I myself have fairly strong representations of articulation, and am able to imagine that I am pronouncing any word whatever, for example 'Constantinople,' with very sharp local sensations, differently located according to the phoneme, while I repeat aloud very quickly and without stopping, a syllable like pa-pa-pa or ti-ti-ti or bro-bro-bro, etc.

greatly with the individual, in spite of the convenient affirmation of the identity of all individuals, which is customary with most clinicians—whose psychological analyses are usually barren enough.[1]

To deny motor types of internal language, and even auditory-motor types which are the most common, while denying kinæsthetic representations, is really to treat well established data[2] a little too cavalierly.

But the assertion that speech is not *conditioned* by kinæsthetic images is on a very different plane.

There is an appearance of contradiction in Dejerine, in that his sub-cortical motor aphasia was an aphemia, with preservation of the motor images. Thus these images would not be sufficient to secure articulation. What would be missing? Their connection with the motor centres. But with what motor centres?

In any case, if the presence of these images were not sufficient, their absence would *ipso facto* involve aphemia; these images would be absolutely necessary.

This is assumed by Bernard-Leroy, who justly criticizes the arguments by which Déjerine establishes the persistence of kinæsthetic images in certain aphemias.[3] And he cites from Saint-Paul's interesting work[4] the observations of Choublier, who, when he

[1] It is, in fact, remarkable that even professed opponents of Dejerine's view, like Moutier, agree with him on this point. In fact, patients suffering from aphasia are generally not recognized and still less analysed before their pathological disorders; and they are often too undeveloped mentally for the analysis to be fruitful; finally, clinical method is satisfied with an approximation sufficient for practical needs.

[2] Moutier, Froment and Monod look for an intellectual representation of the movements of the various muscles involved, which they assume can be discovered by science, and they do not find it. Similarly we do not know, when imagining a movement of the finger or of the arm, what muscles are concerned. The difference is that we can imagine our finger visually, but not our mouth or our larynx, except perhaps in the case of certain speaking deaf-mutes (if the apparent paradox can be excused). The kinæsthetic sensation—or the representation which is only its awakening—is a specific impression, not directly intellectualizable, and localized only roughly in the region of the vocal organs.

[3] *Le langage*, Paris, 1905, pp. 130-142.

[4] Georges Saint-Paul, *Essais sur le langage intérieur*, Paris, 1892, p. 74.

first spoke in public, learned by heart the first part of his speech: "While I was speaking," he says, "it seemed to me that at the moment when my tongue was articulating the phrase I was speaking, I was internally speaking the following phrase, so that, at times, I was afraid of mixing the words of the second phrase with those of the first."

Moreover, the personal observation recorded by Ballet, also cited by Bernard-Leroy, would prove the necessary connection between kinæsthetic representation and verbal articulation. He provoked, by excessive smoking, actual transitory attacks of aphasia, and noted that, when he tried to name objects he could not, though evoking his auditory and visual images, pronounce a word such as 'parapluie': "I endeavoured to co-ordinate the syllables which constituted it," he says, "and while I was articulating very clearly 'parapet' and 'obélisque,' my tongue made a fruitless appeal to my motor memory"; then suddenly while he was fixing his attention on the visual image, the word "burst forth, so to speak, and gushed out"; the motor image was revived by the visual image.[1]

But as a matter of fact, was not the word which "burst forth" pronounced by 'motor habit,' according to the expression of Froment and Monod; suddenly released, without any preliminary awakening of the kinæsthetic representation?

Normally, to have kinæsthetic representation and to be capable of effecting the movement are equivalent; the two terms are so closely linked together that they must both be absent or both be realized at the same time.

But do these ordinary links constitute a necessary connection? It does not seem so. When searching for a word which we cannot remember, we clearly find it because, automatically, we succeed in pronouncing

[1] Gilbert Ballet, *Le langage intérieur et les formes de l'aphasie*, Paris, 1886, pp. 141-142.

it, either by fumbling, or from its context in a phrase or a conversation.

And in this context the remarks of the aphasic doctor Saloz, after his cure, are very instructive: "I often felt," he said, "that I had the syllable or the word in my power, but owing to an unfortunate obstacle, the psychological tracts were suddenly compressed, deranged, obliterated, blocked or perhaps inhibited." A different word might come instead of the word sought. "I am never able," he added, "to tell beforehand whether I can express myself or not. It is a very curious feeling."[1]

Thus the word may or may not be correctly pronounced, without any kinæsthetic representation allowing it either to be seen in advance, or *a fortiori* prepared.

And further, how many verbal automatisms, Pierre Marie's "formulæ of language," true reflexes, arise even among aphemic patients, similar in every way to motor automatisms or congenital reflexes which are by no means necessarily conditioned by a kinæsthetic representation. So we may conclude that images of articulation—which certainly exist as memories of sensations[2] —are not necessary to correct articulation: and it is very improbable that they are sufficient to ensure it; but to this point we shall return later.

In what then does aphemia consist! Is it a paralytic or an ataxic disorder? Pierre Marie and his pupils have never given a precise account of the nature of this motor disorder. Eliminating images—and thereby, they think, memories—they leave undetermined the exact mechanism of the disturbance, which they regard as a simple hindrance in the co-ordination of movements.

In reality everything occurs as if there were loss of

[1] *Cf.* Naville, "Mémoires d'un médecin aphasique," *Archives de Psychologie*, 1918, no 65, pp. 1-57.

[2] We shall consider later the question of the existence of kinæsthetic 'verbal' images distinct from common images.

motor memory, that is to say of the motor habit, the progress of verbal automatism. And this is not a matter of general amnesia or of a diffuse associative disorder.

How, apart from the incito-motor area, which is not itself affected, can there be injury to the acquired mechanisms which allow the correct realization of complex co-ordinated movements? To solve this problem it is necessary to refer to an important idea on which we have already insisted, that of the formation of *co-ordination centres* for complex motor reactions.

Consider the decapitated frog which wipes with its foot a spot on its skin on which a drop of acid has been placed, or a spinal dog (with its spinal cord severed in a high region) which scratches itself when a cutaneous area is slightly stimulated. In these cases, there is a reflex centre which, owing to the action of certain sensory excitations, releases a complex co-ordinated reaction, provoking, in the order desired and with suitable intensities, the operation of the motor cells corresponding to the muscles involved in the action. This operation is prepared; it is controlled by an element which constitutes a centre not, properly speaking, motor, but co-ordinative.

Let us recall again the fine example of a co-ordination centre which is furnished by the movements of the eyes and the head. In order to look to the right or the left, the eyes and the head must make movements of a definite amplitude, with a strict co-ordination of the muscles of both sides. Now looking or turning the head to the right may become impossible in certain lesions which affect the oculogyric centres or the right cephalogyric centres, the 'oculodextrogyric' centre for example, which is situated in the mesencephalon, without any paralysis of the ocular muscles.

The centre will be put into operation, either by retinal impressions (which at the same time can direct the co-ordinated movement of convergence), or by labyrinthine impressions, or by auditory impressions, or again by mnemonic evocation of visual representations, or finally by an impulse of associative origin, by volition. In each of these cases, the incitation which has come by very different tracts will be interpreted by a certain complex reaction released by means of the co-ordination centre which, in communication with the various receptive and central stations, will respond by the prepared reaction which it controls, namely, looking to the right or left.

We may note the similarity between the complex movement of looking to one side or the other, which can be abolished by a lesion that affects only this action in its complexity, without paralysis, and without impairment of the elementary movements of which it is composed, and the enunciation of a word, which requires the operation of a bucco-laryngeal group, under the influence of various excitations, either receptive (reading or repetition) or associative, and which may be abolished without paralysis of the elementary movements necessary—and sufficient—for such enunciation.

Differences exist, however, not only in the number, which is very unequal, of the co-ordinated movements of the process of looking and of articulated language, but more especially in the fact that the centres by means of which we look to the right and left, or up and down, are the pre-established mesencephalic centres that is to say the congenital centres, which are put into operation by a reflex tract, even without the cerebral cortex functioning at all, while the centres of speech are formed by education during the lifetime of the individual—though with a certain hereditary predisposition—and are located in the cortex.[1]

[1] Pierre Marie insists—reacting against Dejerine's view—on this idea of the progressive formation of cortical adaptations. Very young children, affected with right hemiplegia, learn to talk without special difficulties in spite of a lesion of the left hemisphere ("Existe-t-il dans le cerveau humain des centres innés ou préformés de langage," *Presse Médicale*, May 1, 1922, pp. 177-181). The study of dumb children who can hear, such as that de-

The incito-motor centres are themselves co-ordinative. But, when a more complex act requiring a succession of relatively simple acts is repeated very frequently, and becomes automatic, a relay centre is formed, a co-ordinative element, capable of releasing it, by bringing into operation, in the desired order and with the requisite intensity, the various incito-motor elements which control the actions composing the group which makes up the whole automatic activity. This is so especially when numerous analogous actions are possible and may be controlled by very different tracts. We must, indeed, assume this, when we see apraxias abolishing complex habitual automatic acts, and effacing the results of learning, and of progress in skill and rapidity of execution acquired by countless repetitions; and this without paralysis and without impairing the elementary mechanisms. An apraxic patient can no longer aim at anything, make the sign of the cross, blow his nose, or handle his knife and fork, though all the while he recognizes objects and without anæsthesia, paralysis or ataxia; he will behave like a young child who has not yet automatized these mechanisms. There is forgetfulness in this case, but it is due to a localized lesion.[1]

The fact is that this lesion damages the co-ordinative elements—collected in a sort of station analogous to a telephone exchange—which have been specialized by education in the function of bringing into immediate

scribed by André Collin, argues, however, in favour of an hereditary cortical predisposition which would be affected in certain congenital malformations.

[1] There may also be apraxia during great amnesias due to a general disturbance of cerebral functioning, or to demential weakening. But the automatisms of the acts are very resistant; in the great amnesias of certain patients suffering from concussion, due to general injury of the brain, it is only in a short initial phase that we can establish the fact of total apraxias (inability to use a fork or a spoon, to dress oneself, let down one's trousers, etc.) and the recovery always occurs spontaneously, though in many cases no intellectual memory returns for several years (*cf.* Mairet and Piéron, "Les troubles de mémoire d'origine commotionnelle," *Journal de Psychologie*, XII, 4, 1917, pp. 300-328).

operation, as a whole, a group of elementary actions, and the advantage of the education is thus destroyed. When only some one group of co-ordinating elements is affected, some one automatic activity is completely or partially abolished; and these automatic activities that can disappear separately, and have distinct co-ordination centres, include the instrumental execution of the pianist or the violinist, or even of skilled typing, writing and more specially speech.[1]

Among the apraxias, agraphia and aphemia come first. The co-ordination centres of writing and especially of speech are of very great importance, on the one hand, and their disorders cannot be overlooked, and, on the other, the multiplicity of independent complex acts, of written and spoken signs, that they produce, implies a development and a very considerable extension of these centres, which are thenceforward more vulnerable in cerebral lesions; and furthermore, this multiplicity, as a consequence of the resultant competition, prevents —except for a few verbal acts—any deep automatization, and functional disturbances directly affect the most susceptible mechanisms, precisely because of their susceptibility. Education in language consists in the construction of a sort of keyboard, the keys of which must be put into action for the phonemes and phonetic groups which constitute words to be automatically articulated, without fumbling or groping, each key having its connections established with the incito-motor elements of articulation.[2] Injury to these keys, or the

[1] The apraxias abolish complex movements belonging to automatic activities: simple movements are preserved when there are no paralytic disorders. There may also be movements more deeply automatized, whose co-ordination has doubtless become sub-cortical, movements which are repeated in extreme insanity, or in extreme pain when cortical functioning is almost absent. There are no 'amimias' (suppression of the movements of mimicry) in apraxias due to lesions of the cortex, because mimetic automatism is connected with the thalamus.

[2] We know that the incito-motor elements of phonation and of articulation are double, each hemisphere being related to the motor neurones of the bulbar nuclei of both sides. Also the disorders of paralysis of the will, of

M

putting out of use of the keyboard, causes us to lose the whole result of learning to speak, without the motor element being affected.

In this case it is indeed a form of memory which is affected; not, however, the memory of the kinæsthetic impressions of articulation,[1] but the mnemonic constitution of the associative incitor-motor mechanisms, a constitution which, in the course of evolution, as the physiology of the nervous system shows, implies the intervention of the co-ordination centres by a process which we need not be astonished to see produced during the development of the indivdual.

2. *The Phemic Co-ordination Centre*

Just as the ocular co-ordination centres may be put into action by different tracts, of a labyrinthine origin (rotation of the body), auditory (lateral sounds), visual (light suddenly appearing in the periphery of the field), volitional (for the explanation of the field), or imaginative (evocation of a lateral image), so the centre of phemic co-ordination, or rather one of the relay stations of this complex centre, can be put into action by auditory (repetition) or visual (reading aloud) impressions, by tendencies, feelings and sensory images (spontaneous expression, emotional reaction, naming of objects, etc.)

phonation and articulation—true anarthria or accentuated dysarthria—appear only in double hemiplegias with lesions extending to the lower part of the ascending frontal or to the bundles which proceed from it (the clinical type of the paralysis known as 'pseudo-bulbar' because it has long been confused with the labio-glosso-laryngeal paralysis due to the lesion of the motor nuclei of the bulb on the area of the last pairs of cranial nerves).

[1] This is a physiological conception (S. Exner's 'Senso-mobilität') which has been regarded by many able writers as a necessity, even for the simple incito-motor function of the cortex—which is already co-ordinative, as we have seen—in kinæsthetic memory. It owed its origin to a confusion of the sensory centres and the incito-motor centres of the cortex, yet these centres, although closely connected, are absolutely independent and distinct in function. Surely kinæsthetic images will not for ever be invoked to explain reflex movements of looking at objects and their loss will not always account for the peculiar apraxia which consists in the suppression of the power of looking to the right or left through a mesencephalic lesion!

and even by the mnemonic evocation of corresponding auditory, visual, or kinæsthetic impressions, or finally by the phenomena of associative irradiation that are referred to as ideas.[1]

To sum up: audition of a word, or auditory memory; vision of a word, or visual memory; memory of the articulation of a word; perception, by one sensory tract or by several, of an object of which the word is the symbol; associative expression of feelings or of ideas: —these are the essential means utilized in the activation of the phemic centre. One or other of the categories usually employed may predominate. In the case of an imbecile, repetition without comprehension, psittacism, may prevail; the rôle of visual impressions is null or nearly so among the illiterate; the deaf from birth who have learned to speak have no auditory impressions to intervene. But, normally, it is feelings and ideas that appear in action, in the form of language.

Let us suppose that localized lesions succeed in interrupting one of the tracts which give access to the phemic centre. Just as the suppression of the connection between the vestibular or cochlear nuclei and the centre for direction of vision involve the suppression of reflexes of labyrinthine or auditory origin, so the interruption of the association paths—included in the arcuate bundle—which connect the auditory area and the centre of phemic co-ordination, will prevent the repetition. It will prevent it completely in the case of unknown phonemes, of words in a foreign language which has not been learned; it should not prevent it in

[1] Local irritation may also set in operation phemic impulses, besides hallucinatory representations or certain convulsive movements, in Jacksonian epilepsy. I have had frequent occasion to observe slight attacks of epileptic vertigo in the case of a man who suddenly checked himself in the middle o an act, grew pale, blushed, and repeated several times in a fit of complete absent-mindedness: "Shut up? Well, shut up then," of course without preserving any memory of these verbal convulsions. In echolalia—the prolonged and involuntary repetition of words or phrases—a spasmodic form of speech occurs (Trénel and Crinon) which often accompanies spasmodic laughter or speech.

the case of known and understood words, for the evocation of a visual representation or of intellectual associations will allow indirect action on the phemic centre and ensure the enunciation of the word whose direct repetition is impossible.

For this to occur, the other mechanisms of evocation must not have been affected, spontaneous speech must be correct, writing to dictation, reading and comprehension must be unimpaired.

Sometimes, however, all the conditions are obviously present and yet the repetition of a word, spontaneously pronounced in a correct fashion, is impossible. This is a curious phenomenon which I noted in one of my aphasic war patients.

It is explained by the fact that, in such a case, with functional disorders (continuous amnesia or aprosexia), the compulsory repetition distracts the attention, and demands an effort—though a vain one—preventing the associative evocation which would ensure comprehension.[1]

When attention is brought to bear on the phoneme, and is not allowed to wander to the associative automatism which is characteristic of recognition, it is remarkable that the word seems strange like a word from an unknown language. If I hear as a sound the phonemes *ban—ur*—they do not seem to have any relationship to the word *banner*, which I understand almost without hearing it, without, that is to say, noticing its auditory characteristics. My patient, who was capable of naming an object and yet unable to repeat the name of the object when asked to do so, was the victim of a deviation of attention of this sort, which, as a result of his functional injury, completely debarred the mechanism of evocation by association paths.

These circumstances are rarely found in conjunction, and we have scarcely any examples of verbal deafness

[1] There is a similar mechanism which may explain optical or tactile aphasia, when the perception of an object—with recognition—no longer evokes the corresponding word.

preventing repetition but not comprehension. It is generally the reverse which occurs, but we shall return to this point.

The phemic centre may then be isolated in relation to one of the centres capable of acting on it; sometimes spontaneous speech is impossible owing to a disturbance of the associative area in its relations with the phemic centre, and servile repetition continues.

Usually, in aphemias, whatever may be the tract employed for putting the co-ordination centre into operation, the check is the same, for either all the tracts have been interrupted before reaching the centre, or the centre itself has been destroyed by the lesion, or again the connections of the centre with the incito-motor elements have been broken. It is impossible to differentiate the type of destruction in a case of complete aphemia. When the aphemia is partial and all the tracts of access give like results, this is because the lesion bears on the keys of the co-ordinative keyboard or on its organs of motor transmission. If the keys of a typewriter are broken, or out of order, or if they no longer act when struck, the corresponding letters will be lacking in the written text.

In incomplete aphemia, we sometimes find paraphemia, that is to say, in speech some words are pronounced in place of others. If there is no intellectual disorder to explain it, what has occurred is a deviation of connections. An injury to the association bundles which lead to the phemic centre, destroying the isolation of the fibres like an entanglement in the wires of a telephonic system, a disorder of chronaxies, a confusion of syntonies, will account for this more or less accentuated phenomenon which, in a mild form, may proceed solely from a certain inattention in speech.[1]

[1] When thought goes quicker than speech, new ideas seek expression and involve corresponding words which are inserted among the terms relating to the preceding ideas, combining with them and distorting them. This is especially true in writing. We may or may not notice it ourselves.

A disturbance of the actual keys of the keyboard at the stage of realization is capable also of producing deviations or slips, involving paraphemia, especially when the keys are highly sensitive and their operation is rendered easier by automatism. Almost all aphemic patients when trying to talk succeed in pronouncing monosyllables ('yes' or 'no'), formulæ which constitute true verbal reflexes—oaths, for example, which have become the means of expressing emotion.

The destruction of the phemic centre or the disorganization of its organs of motor transmission has not been so complete as to make it impossible for certain very automatic mechanisms to survive.

Thus a worn-out typewriter sometimes succeeds in writing one letter—always the same one.

When several languages are spoken, they correspond to distinct keyboards, and—in exceptional cases—may be selectively injured. Generally it is the least automatic which, in ordinary lesions, are the first to be impaired in their functioning.

3. *The Graphic Co-ordination Centre*

In spite of Dejerine's arguments there is nothing to justify our discarding the idea of the formation of a co-ordination centre for graphic mechanisms become automatic, as well as for habitual and complex praxias, such as speech. If there were an hereditary predisposition to phemic co-ordination—and we can in fact assume it—this is only realized, as Pierre Marie contends, in the course of individual development. And though it is not all men who write, even speech is lacking in uneducated deaf-mutes. We can write with a machine, but we should also talk with a machine if the sounds could be given out mechanically by tapping the keys corresponding to the phonemes, as we talk by signs to a deaf-mute or in semaphoring.

It is true that we can write with the left hand or with the arm and the foot, as we should draw, when we cannot make use of the trained right hand; but the right hand, when not paralysed, is in the same case as the left hand when it loses the benefit of its acquired automatisms. It can draw and even draw from memory, if the visual representations are available—which is not always the case even without verbal blindness—but it cannot achieve automatic execution, the realization in writing of an idea or of phonemes corresponding to well-known words which have often been written.

This localized loss of motor writing-memories is again the result of an injury, either in the structure itself or in its connections, to the centre where the co-ordinating stations which are constituted during the progress of the graphic habit are juxtaposed.

Pure agraphia, which is rarer than aphemia, is certainly found, generally without injury of the function of language, during the regression of more complex disorders, but showing the possibility of an isolated disorder of these mechanisms.

The question at issue is not whether kinæsthetic representations are abolished—they may persist, it seems, in certain agraphias—but whether the co-ordination of automatic graphic movements is still possible.

Visual representations are not necessary for writing, since the blind learn free-hand writing, although the relations between graphism and vision are normally as close as those between speech and hearing.

In pseudo-agraphia due to pure verbal blindness, we are dealing with ill-educated individuals who have scarcely any knowledge of writing, have not automatized or formed a co-ordination centre for it, and who must draw the model imagined from the constituent letters of the words. They do this a little better with the more skilful hand than with the other, but are checked when they forget the representations which they are copying. Verbal blindness does not prevent the automatisms from operating—in spite of the impossibility of re-reading—when education has set up a graphic co-ordination centre. A very clear case of this has come under my observation.[1]

The keys of the co-ordinative keyboard may also be selectively affected; it being impossible to write certain words, and as a rule these may be any words.[2] Figures have a co-ordinative keyboard near, but distinct from, that of words and letters. As a rule agraphic patients write them correctly, but sometimes they cannot. There are even distinct keys for numbers equivalent to numerical words, at least for certain numbers (the year of birth, for example; numbers with a symbolic significance, such as 1870, etc.), so that these numbers are still correctly written when other figures or numbers cannot be managed.

Sometimes numbers, although correctly understood, are faultily written, though the digits are correct and the assembling of separate signs by means of vision is correct; and this without any other disorder of writing.[3]

4. *The Idea of the Sensory Verbal Image and Receptive Co-ordination Centres*

The Agnosias

In order to understand verbal deafness and verbal blindness, a loss of auditory and visual images of words has been invoked. But the idea of a sensory verbal image, though it does not imply the greater confusion

[1] In this case, an attempt at design-writing by copying the graphic signs was impossible with the left hand. There may, however, be an imitation with the left hand of represented movements of the right hand, thanks to the recall of kinæsthetic impressions, and this imitation will occur symmetrically, that is to say, mirror-wise.

[2] In some cases it is impossible to write certain letters, whereas in the words which contain them they are correctly formed: the key corresponding to the isolated letter is affected, but there are keys for the words and certain of them still function.

[3] Otto Sittig, "Über Störungen des Ziffernschreibens bei Aphasischen," *Zeitschrift für Pathopsychologie*, 1917, III, pp. 298-396. Several cephalic patients write numbers of two digits in reverse order.

of the motor image, has not always been accepted and has not even been clearly formulated.

In his interesting work on language, Eugène Bernard-Leroy criticizes the idea in the following words:

"The first interpretation which comes to mind is that the authors mean by a verbal image the memory of the auditory perception of a word; but two objections can be raised to this conception. The first is that this memory is not an image; we must conceive of it as a complex including an image, emotions, etc., and having as a centre the auditory sensation itself. It is a system which tends to develop; it is a view of the mind as a whole, a realized abstraction, for this system only has reality in so far as it develops. The second objection is that there is no 'lost' or 'effaced' memory. If the memory of a word, especially, were lost, the patient would no longer have any perception of this word. As a matter of fact, he has a crude or even a differentiated perception of it.

"But perhaps what is meant by the expression, verbal images, is the images, emotions, etc., in short, the states of consciousness that constitute the system habitually connected with the audition of the word. This second interpretation does not render the theory any more acceptable. If these states of consciousness were destroyed or even if the links which inter-connect them were broken and the system dissociated, this system could not in any case appear. In order that it may be evoked in a perfectly normal way, however, it is enough for the word to be read instead of being heard, if it is a matter of verbal deafness, or heard instead of being read, if it is a matter of verbal blindness.

"It is precisely this last consideration which leads us to the interpretation, purely psychological of course, that what is impaired and disordered is the association between the perception of the word, visual in one case, auditory in the other, and the system of images that it must evoke. Both terms continue, but the chain which united them is broken; the appearance of the first no longer involves the appearance of the second."[1]

The substitution, for the loss of sensory images, of an associative, intellectual, injury, to explain verbal deafness and blindness, characterizes Pierre Marie's conception, according to which aphasia—of a single clinical variety only—is only a lack of comprehension of language. Moutier too adopts Bernard-Leroy's critique. "It is the interpretation of the image and not the image itself that is lacking,"[2] he writes; but going further, he carries his criticism of the notion of an image in general to the point of complete negation. He cannot separate the image of the words from the thought. "To sum up, these thoughts, the words, and these abstractions, the images, from an indissoluble whole in which no element is distinct."[3] And after considering the various conceptions of the image, and refusing it the rôle of a cerebral stereotype or schema, and that of an *idée-force*, he excludes it definitively: "The image is a word: we cannot define it, we can only find to what it corresponds; it is a simple façade behind which nothing goes on."[4]

This view is certainly too extreme: when we dream that we hear someone speaking to us, that we are seeing him move, or when we imagine ourselves to be running, we have a representation involving visual, auditory, and kinæsthetic images as well as mnemonic reproductions of perceptions, sometimes combined so as to form new aspects. The image is thus a datum of common sense, whose exact nature and mechanism alone are open to discussion.

It is not difficult, given a certain capacity for visual imagination, to imagine a page from a book with the words we have read there: we can imagine the voice of a friend pronouncing a phrase. We thus have visual and auditory images which are verbal images.

[1] *Le Langage*, pp. 83-84.
[2] *L'aphasie de Broca*, p. 245.
[3] *Ibid.*, p. 239.
[4] *Ibid.*, p. 244.

The existence of verbal images cannot be denied.[1] But this does not imply that verbal deafness and blindness are due to the loss of auditory or visual images of words, nor that there is a special centre forming a sort of storehouse for these images. These hypotheses are, in fact, unsatisfying, and are open to many criticisms and lines of attack.

Let us look more closely at what constitutes the evocation of an image.

It is childish to suppose that the brain constitutes a storehouse where little stereotypes are deposited, photographic images of events which have affected the senses, and that memory serves to bring them eventually to light. The mnemonic awakening of a sensation, in which the peculiar property of the image resides, is the setting in operation, through an association path, of the receptive sensory elements which have been drawn into action by peripheral stimulation. Let us assume that I provoke the visual image of a printed page—taking such an example because visual images give the very best illusion of being pictures or photographic prints—it is certain that I can see the whole page distinctly in my imagination, and with an intensity capable of many degrees; I can evoke a white mass of rectangular form with greyish lines as though I had an instantaneous floating vision of the page. If I wish to read, I shall successively evoke distinct impressions, very limited in extent, of words or small groups of words, with a representation of the movement of visual exploration along the lines. Moreover, from a mass of words I should be able to imagine one word in isolation. When I have seen this word, the different retinal elements receiving impressions of high or low luminosity bring into play the central elements which correspond to them respectively, and produce simultaneous sensations of white and black which constitute

[1] Froment and Monod, who reject the motor image, consider that the reality of auditory and visual verbal images cannot be doubted; *loc. cit.*

the frame or design of the word. The fully successful and complete evocation of this design is the activation, this time centrally initiated, of the same cortical receptive elements whose topography corresponds to the peripheral elements of the retinal macula, with the same relative intensity, resulting in black and white. To imagine that there is a storehouse for the visual images of words, distinct from other visual images, is to flout the evidence of neurology; such a conception was permissible for the Epicureans, but hardly for the man of science to-day! Criticism of the idea of a verbal image as a distinct entity is therefore fully justified. Images are the mnemonic processes of the awakening of sensations; there may then be images of words; but nothing distinguishes them in the first analysis from other images, in their dynamic realization.

We cannot lose the power of evoking images belonging to one sense without losing that of evoking the corresponding verbal images, but the facts show that we can lose the evocation of the verbal images alone. This means that the mechanisms of evoking these images are affected. An associative process no longer functions as before. But we cannot say that the verbal images, although not evocable, are preserved, because the image has no existence outside the process of evocation of the elementary sensory traces; the image is the congeries of evocative processes which activate as a specific whole elements serving for every possible combination: the order of the successive phonemes constitutes the auditory image of a word, the same phonemes in another order giving another word.

Thus it is not the utilization of a stereotype image which is injured, but the realization of the image, an associative dynamism. Nor may we regard the incapacity to evoke verbal images as a purely intellectual disorder; we are really dealing with a sensory evocation but one whose mechanism is associative and for that very reason intellectual.

And if, under this dynamic aspect of a congeries of associations that evoke elementary sensory data, we imagine the verbal image, we can again say that verbal deafness or blindness consists in the loss of the auditory or visual images of the words.

But how can this selective loss of the evocative dynamisms occur? In disorders bearing on the association paths, the images of objects would have to be lacking as well as the images of words, the confused representation of the page and the grey lines as well as the distinct successive representation of the words which form the lines. This is not so.

If, therefore, a limited lesion selectively suppresses the power of evoking on its behalf the auditory or visual representations of words, we are justified in holding that this is due to the educative formation of a relay station, of a central co-ordinating station. Just as, in thought, the enunciation of a word occurs by means of the phemic co-ordination centre, so the auditory or visual evocation of that word requires also an analysing and distributing apparatus which, under influences arising from various sources, releases the excitations—in suitable order, with the desired relative intensities—no longer of incito-motor elements corresponding to the actions involved in the articulation of the word, but of receptive elements of the receptive region involved in the auditory, visual, and kinæsthetic realization of this word.

But unlike the motor co-ordination centres which function only in one direction, the sensory co-ordination centres which must be in evidence in this evocation of verbal images of an associative origin, have also an inverse rôle, which may even be regarded as their principal rôle; they evoke the manifold associations involved by comprehension, beginning with the images aroused peripherally, that is to say beginning with perceptions. And we can readily understand that a co-ordination centre may be necessary for the auditory or visual comprehension of language. When so many words, whose sensory groups may be so close together, are endowed with such different evocative powers and involve such varied significations, we can imagine the complexity of the association paths which must directly connect the many receptive elements involved—in the visual area, for example—not only one with another, but with the auditory receptive elements (for the auditory evocation of the word seen); and also with all the elements on which depend the feelings, attitudes and reactions implicated in this comprehension, and with all the receptive elements of all the sensory areas that ensure the evocation of the various images that the sense of the word may allow![1]

As well suppose that if all the inhabitants of Paris had telephones and communicated with one another, they would have to have separate wires connecting each one with all the others. We should then have to assume that, if groups were formed, when one group communicated with another, simultaneously all the members of the first group would have to be put into connection with one another, and each of them with all the members of the other group, who would themselves be inter-connected. We find in nature processes of simplification analogous to those which man has contrived in like cases.

The formation of central stations intermediate between one sensory area and the others is evidently one of the characteristics of cerebral functioning. Thanks to these relays, a word, for which a key has been secured—or even several keys which can be used by substitution on the keyboard[2]—when it is seen or heard, enters

[1] Sollier, in view of the multiplicity of the paths here implied, thinks it impossible that one image can be individually united to all the images that it is capable of evoking. And he seeks a solution of the problem in a conception of the image as a dynamic state of an entire centre (*Essai critique et théorique sur l'association*, 1907). But the existence of co-ordinating levels clearly disposes of the difficulty.

[2] When we speak several languages and have prepared ourselves to follow one of them, and it is another which is spoken, we have the feeling that it is necessary to 'turn over the page,' to change the register, especially if the

into correspondence with this key, with which the sensory complex is connected. From this point there start associative impulses in prepared tracts towards the co-ordinating phemic or graphic centres which allow repetition or writing, towards the other sensory co-ordination centres, which ensure the evocation of the various images of the word, towards the groups which form images of objects or memories of events, and towards the affective or motor centres—awakening feelings, tendencies, attitudes, reactions, etc., according to the mnemonic preparation of the association paths, and according to the sensibilizing influence of the mental orientation, of the momentary environment, of the immediately previous events, etc.[1]

An injury to the relays or the communicative tracts of these relays with their sensory areas, or finally to the association bundles which emanate from them, will produce the disorders characteristic of sensory aphasia, partial or complete, verbal deafness or verbal blindness. And their similarity to the aphemias is remarkable.

Aphemia and agraphia are particular forms of apraxia. Verbal deafness or blindness—which consists in a lack of comprehension of the auditory or visual images of words, and in an incapacity to utilize them or interpret them by speech or writing—are particular forms of agnosia. And in fact there are non-verbal agnosias which are sometimes called asymbolias.[2] Thus psychic

same word appears with a different signification in the two idioms. And in our own language there are homonyms which have distinct pegs in different regions of the keyboard. The '*leaves* of a printed book' have one individuality, requiring a separate corresponding co-ordinator, and the '*leaves* of a tree' have another.

[1] As a result of experimental research on association, in 1904, I was led to show the complexity of the factors governing evocation (*cf.* "La conception générale de l'association et les données de l'expérience," *Revue Philosophique*, 1904, pp. 493-518). And I have often insisted since then on this essential idea, in opposition to the simple schema of linear associative connection (*cf.* for example *l'Evolution de la Mémoire*, 1910, p. 234).

[2] The symbolic character of objects, and the perceptual significance which this involves, is in fact abolished. The term asymbolia is generally confined to agnosia of signs. But all objects, from a certain point of view, are signs.

blindness is characterized by failure to recognize objects perceived. In verbal blindness, the words are not understood, but graphic characters as such are; in psychic blindness, writing itself is not recognized.

When the sight of objects no longer involves the habitual associative evocations, there are, in the handling of these objects, incoherences which may remind us of apraxic or demential disorders.

Noises, which are attributed to well-defined causes—so that in verbal deafness if the terms of a language are not understood, the language as such is at least identified—lose all meaning in psychic deafness.

We also find cases of tactile agnosia, in which, without marked sensory disorders, objects felt no longer awaken either the idea of their nature and use or the word which designates them. And in the case of the blind, reading with their fingers, a tactile agnosia of words, a verbal anæsthesia, is conceivable.

Apraxias and agnosias correspond very closely to the two poles of mental life, which proceeds from the reception of external stimuli in the direction of reactions to the physical and social environment.

5. *The Auditory Co-ordination Centre*

It can be readily understood that disorders in the functioning of the relay stations, which ensure characteristic evocations of words or groups of words that are the object of common verbal experiences, prevent comprehension; repetition is generally less affected in incomplete injuries, but may be affected separately. In this case, the bundle which connects the auditory and phemic co-ordination centres is separately interrupted, organically or functionally. Of course, if there is a diminution of associative functioning, an intellectual injury, comprehension may be more or less abolished without the co-ordination centre being necessarily impaired; repetition is still possible, which proves its integrity.

In general disorders of unequal intensity the same law holds throughout. The most automatized and most usual expressions are the most tenacious, and can survive separately in the wreck of auditory comprehension: the patient's name is generally recognized. On the other hand, grammatical forms and the significance of syntax are forgotten first, and the prominent words alone are understood.

Little-used foreign languages are generally very fragile.

But selective lesions may have apparently capricious consequences, and the comprehension of certain categories of words or of a language which is not the one least used, may alone be affected.

On the other hand, an extension of verbal deafness may occur in the form of psychic deafness, and musical deafness in particular sometimes accompanies it.[1]

In incomplete verbal deafness we often find confusions which, when they depend on paraphasias of expression, or on paraphemias, are true paraphasias of comprehension, or paragnosias. In one of my own cases I got examples of a form of paragnosia constituting verbal paracousia: the patient put his thumb in his mouth when asked to put his little finger in his left ear.[2] The word heard no longer evokes the corresponding associations, but, if it does not damage the appropriate key of the co-ordinative keyboard, it may yet

[1] The association of words with music in songs appears to be close enough for a totally aphasic patient to be able to understand and repeat a song, and to pronounce the words correctly, provided that he sings it, though language is not understood and speech is impossible—a good example of a functional dissociation implying an anatomical independence of co-ordinating keyboards (*cf.* L. Bianchi, "La fonction musicale du cerveau et sa localisation," *Scientia*, 1922, XVI, pp. 25-36).

[2] In a very similar case, a patient, whose verbal deafness was growing less marked, pointed to his teeth when asked to point to his tongue, or to his moustache instead of his hair (*cf.* A. Pick, *Ueber das Sprachverständnis*, 1909).

reach the part of the keyboard where that key occurs and act on its neighbours, causing analogous reactions. Sometimes one word is taken for another word which sounds the same and is better known; and this is only the exaggeration of a normal fact, the popular assimilation of the less usual with the more usual, involving linguistic deformations which are very often noticed.

Verbal deafness is also accompanied by the incapacity to evoke, according to the sense, the auditory image of the corresponding words. If this disorder is isolated, speech may remain correct: but we frequently observe phenomena of paraphasia, due to the absence of auditory control, and perhaps preparation of speech by auditory evocation. Certainly, in such cases, the form of thought, more or less kinæsthetic or auditory, should play some part, though this, in the absence of adequate preliminary knowledge of the patient, may be difficult to establish. In fact, in spite of verbal deafness, paraphasic patients may perceive their errors and correct them, making use of kinæsthetic impressions; and there are paraphasic patients who, without suffering from verbal deafness, do not perceive them.[1]

Verbal deafness, as such, is therefore a factor which favours paraphasia, the mechanism of which can be due to distractions, phemic disorders or associative or intellectual disturbances, but it is not sufficient to produce it and has not the necessary connection with it.

If, however, auditory control is not absolutely indispensable for the articulation of words,[2] because of the part which may be played by kinæsthetic control—and in this connection, patients deaf from birth who have

[1] In norma paraphasia errors are often not perceived and are not corrected.

[2] It is surprising to find Bernheim declaring—and with the approval of Moutier—that in verbal deafness there are certainly acoustic images since speech persists: the patient can talk, "that is to say, he can find the words he needs: the acoustic image of these words and their significance is therefore not abolished" (Bernheim, *Doctrine de l'aphasie, Conception nouvelle*, 1907). If acoustic images were absolutely necessary for speech it would be futile to attempt to teach deaf-mutes. But this is not the case.

learned to speak furnish a conclusive example—it seems to be absolutely indispensable for singing, for the giving out of sounds of regular tonality: musical deafness makes singing without false notes impossible.

The graduated melody of language—which is not as a rule affected in verbal deafness, but is lacking in deaf-mutes—perhaps needs an auditory control which does not seem to be connected with verbal audition. There is here, among Europeans, a form of mimicry, of expression of feeling. But when, as in Chinese, the word requires for its verbal specification and for its symbolic value a tonal utterance of a certain kind, we may wonder whether pure verbal deafness would or would not involve disorders of speech from the point of view of this essentially verbal melody. We lack, in this connection, analysed observations of aphasia among the Chinese, and *a fortiori*, observations of that clinical rarity, pure verbal deafness.

6. *The Visual Co-ordination Centre*

The parallelism of function between the visual and auditory co-ordination centres is complete, at least in the case of a literate individual who has acquired the automatism of reading.

As in verbal deafness, it is comprehension which, in incomplete verbal blindness, is first impaired and last recovered; reading aloud, through action on the phemic centre, is less fragile.[1]

It seems that there is no dissociation between comprehension and the capacity of auditory evocation in pure verbal blindness: this is because, if the auditory evocation worked well, it would involve *ipso facto*—in the absence of verbal deafness—comprehension.

[1] In studying pure verbal blindness, during recovery, with re-education, I found that reading aloud—in spite of difficulties due to the dispersion of attention necessitated by the phemic effort—permitted an indirect comprehension, the visual representation of words being transformed, by means of speech, into an auditory or kinæsthetic representation, retaining the power of co-ordinated evocation.

In certain cases even it is possible that comprehension comes about normally through the bringing into action of elements of the auditory co-ordination centre in connection with the visual centre.

This is certainly not a universal fact, since there are a few cases of pure verbal deafness. But it may be suggested that the rarity of these cases results in part from this process of visual comprehension and perhaps also of phemic or graphic interpretation, *by means of* auditory representation: if the latter were made impossible by an injury to its co-ordination centre, reading itself could no longer occur.

It is probable, however, that the principal reason for the association of verbal blindness and verbal deafness lies in the proximity of the co-ordination centres, and in the topography of the arterial irrigation, the usual circulatory disorders affecting at the same time both co-ordinating areas. Moreover, this association also involves deeper disorders, as we shall see when we come to consider Wernicke's aphasia. Like verbal deafness, which affects the least known languages before it bears on the mother tongue, partial alexia also prevents, at first, the comprehension of complete phrases, or of verbs in their grammatical form, with mood and tense. The prominent words are recognized and the patient guesses and constructs a meaning out of these words.

The comprehension of words—and especially of the words most often read—outlasts the recognition of syllables and letters with persons who have had great practice in reading.[1]

The hierarchy of disorders according to the degree of verbal blindness is very regular: but there are also

[1] Cases have even been published of pure letter-blindness with preservation of the reading of words, because, as G. Ballet and Laignel-Lavastine have correctly remarked, in the case of a cultivated individual reading of the word has become synthetic—and we know that it is so from the first in certain methods of reading such as that of Decroly, and that the word is recognized by its general outline.

partial and irregular injuries due to the fact that certain keys only of the co-ordinative keyboard, or certain parts of the keyboard, are destroyed or warped. There will be certain words which are not read, or numbers only, or only a customary language. Musical blindness—the inability to comprehend musical signs—which usually accompanies verbal blindness, may be distinct from it.[1]

Verbal blindness may be one aspect of a more extended psychic blindness.[2] In ordinary cases, symbols (playing cards, a flag, etc.) are recognized, and objects are correctly named. And this fact shows the specialization of recognition of graphic signs, the distinct seat and the vulnerability of the co-ordination centre involved.

But, as we have already said, a very rare curiosity may occur, an optical aphasia without verbal blindness, an incapacity to name objects, in spite of recognition and correct use. We have here a fact which corresponds to the isolated incapacity to repeat speech heard though comprehension is preserved. For such a disorder to appear, we require on the one hand the breaking of a single association bundle—in this case a bundle linking to the verbal co-ordination centres the gnosic co-ordination centre serving as a relay in the recognition of common objects — without lesion of the centre itself, for if this were affected there would be complete psychic blindness ; and at the same time a disorder of attention, impairing recognition, in the effort to get

[1] Here again there are differences which may be connected as in the ordinary case with the degree of perturbation, the better acquired automatisms being the most resistant : reading in the key of F disappears before reading of the key of C and reappears after it. And there are others connected by chance with the distribution of very limited lesions.

[2] Thus Faure-Beaulieu and Jacquet record a case of pure verbal blindness in the course of the regression of a complete visual agnosia : the patient, at the outset, could no longer recognize objects or the place she was in, and was continually getting lost ; after a little there remained only a limited alexia, and the reading of figures returned as well as the ability to tell the time ("Alexie pur, reliquat d'agnosie visuelle," *Revue Neurologique*, 1924, XXXI (11), pp. 495-499).

the name, so that it could not be indirectly found by the play of intellectual associations which constitute recognition.

As in incomplete verbal deafness, we frequently find in incomplete verbal blindness, or paragnosia, a verbal 'paranopsia,' or paralexia: one word is taken for another and understood wrongly. Generally the error is connected with an analogy of form—a more usual word being substituted for the word really seen[1]—but sometimes it is connected with the fact that disorders of the keys of the keyboard or of the association paths involve confusion, so that, in the same part of the keyboard, neighbouring keys of analogous significance are brought into action by the reading.

We cited above, as an example of auditory paragnosia, the patient who put his thumb in his mouth when asked to put his little finger in his left ear. This patient also exhibited paralexia. Given the written order: "Get up and go round the table," he would get up and close the drawer of the table.

We shall not return to these connections between verbal blindness and agraphia, or to the influence of visual images in writing; these images are not necessary, since the blind may learn to write by kinetic and tactile means. But the control of vision, which is important for the realization of automatisms,[2] remains

[1] This is another case of the exaggeration of a normal phenomenon. In rapid reading a more usual word is frequently taken for a less usual word when a sense remains possible. Proof-readers and copyists provide examples of this daily. This common paralexia occurs in one of Moutier's cases (obs. XXXIX) who when dealing with the word *main* (hand), to show that he understood, drew *pain* (loaf of bread).

[2] In a case of paralysis of the right hand, if there is no kinetic transfer to the left hand—which implies symmetrical mirror-writing—the writing of the left hand becomes a copy of visual representations (and kinetic ocular representations), as in the case of a hemiplegic patient affected by aphemia and incomplete verbal blindness, who drew with his left hand large typographical capitals, that is to say the shapes of the best known letters: in free-hand he produced mirror-writing (*cf.* Ch. Nicolle and A. Halipré, "L'écriture en miroir: cécité verbale pure et centre de l'agraphie," *Presse médicale*, April 20, 1895, pp. 148-139).

useful in preventing paragraphia or the orthographic errors sometimes found in the writing of educated patients affected with verbal blindness and preserving graphic automatism intact: the impossibility of re-reading prevents corrections. But the normal individual who does not re-read is liable to make similar mistakes.

7. *The Problem of Kinæsthetic Co-ordination Centres*

As we have already shown, there can be no doubt about the existence of kinæsthetic images corresponding to the articulation of words. That these representations of movements may play a rôle in speech, but that this rôle is not indispensable, and, in particular, that there is a balance between auditory and kinæsthetic evocations, is also an obvious inference from certain facts which we have adduced.

But whether there is a verbal co-ordination centre which ensures a certain autonomy to kinæsthetic images of language as well as to visual and auditory images, is an intricate problem and one which is by no means solved.

Let us assume that in certain very limited lesions there may be suppression of verbal kinæsthetic images without articulatory anæsthesia; the kinæsthetic evocation of words would then be impossible through the association paths and the impressions felt during speech would not by themselves be sufficient for compression. But these disturbances would not be manifest, even if thought were carried on solely by the aid of kinæsthetic images of words; and this certainly does not often occur, since auditory images always play some part; it would be enough to speak one's thought in a whisper, and to hear it, for all difficulty to vanish. And, on the other hand, we do not in practice recognize words by the sensations of our own articulation: we hear them.

Thus this disorder, if it occurred, might well not be

noticed by the patient and might remain unknown. And in particular, the probable proximity of the kinæsthetic co-ordination centre and of the phemic co-ordination centre would make it very difficult for the former to be injured without the latter being affected.

In actual fact, there is no evidence of pure verbal kinetic anæsthesia. But in the case of Saloz, the aphasic doctor who recovered and left some interesting memoirs, we find that the complete absence of kinæsthetic representations coincided with a very incomplete aphemia: words were correctly pronounced although it was never possible to know in advance whether they would be, as their representative kinetic evocation did not occur.[1]

Moreover, from the fact of the partial association of aphemia and from the loss of the power of imagining the articulation of words,[2] we may infer a centre of verbal kinæsthetic co-ordination, in close connection with the phemic co-ordination centre, but without the confusion involved in the inadmissible idea of a motor image found in the text-books.

Sensory impressions and representations of movement certainly have a considerable influence on motor execution: when a child learns to use its limbs, the success of an act becomes associated with certain kinæsthetic impressions which will be used later to direct the repetition of that act. And kinæsthetic evocation has a strong tendency, as a result of close association, to provoke motor objectivation.

[1] Kinæsthetic evocation enables us to imagine a movement in advance: the jumper imagines himself above the bar, in representing to himself the possibility of success.

[2] Cases of this would be frequent if, with Dejerine, and his pupils, we were to grant conclusive value to the Proust-Lichtheim test and similar tests; if in aphemias—regarded in that case as sub-cortical—where the patient can indicate the number of letters or syllables of a word which he cannot pronounce, we were to assume the integrity of the kinæsthetic images of inner speech. But it is too evident that the success of these tests establishes only, in the case of a fairly well educated individual, the preservation of visual or auditory or also perhaps—but not certainly—kinæsthetic images.

But, with speech, auditory sensations also occur in the normal case—kinæsthesia alone, after the temporary aid of mirror-vision, governing articulation in the educated deaf-mute—and the success of the verbal act becomes associated not only with impressions of articulation and of phonation, but also with sound-impressions. And as we have said, with regard to singing, the auditory impression, unaided, is delicate enough to ensure effective control. So an auditivo-kinæsthetic group tends to be formed for motor regulation. Auditory representation tends to provoke articulation and kinæsthetic representation, just as the latter arouses movement and is irradiated in an auditory "echo of thought";[1] and finally, speech gives rise to kinæsthetic and auditory impressions at the same time.

It is, then, normal that 'internal speech,' the evocation of words, should generally occur in an auditivo-kinæsthetic form, often with the outline of a real articulation, and a marked predominance on the auditory or the kinæsthetic side; articulation, the outline of the motor objectivation, admitting of many degrees.[2]

The auditivo-kinæsthetic group is generally so compact and the reciprocal evocation is produced with such force that it is difficult to analyse impressions; and this difficulty of analysis appears when we interrogate anyone affected with verbal hallucinations: he hears the voices which speak to him, he hears the words distinctly, but these voices are localized in his throat or his chest.[3] There are kinæsthetic impressions, usually reinforced

[1] This "echo of thought" is the actual expression used by Egger, for whom the auditory representation in internal language was decidedly predominant.

[2] It is none the less true that certain cultivated persons can use visual images, and can even use these images in preference to others.

[3] The weakness of the auditory evocation does not lead to a sufficiently sharp objectivation and as the attitude of listening is not taken, localization occurs where there are confused impressions which attract the attention. Certain persons *hear* their inner speech in their chests normally, as did Bourdon, whose auto-observation is reported by Saint-Paul (*Le Langage intérieur*, p. 93).

by a real outline of articulation, as the apparatus of the phonetician can prove—with the habitual localization of these impressions—and at the same time a faint and indistinct auditory echo; or there is an auditory evocation which involves phemic repetition and, in any case, kinæsthetic representation; or again a phemic automatism will give rise to the auditivo-kinæsthetic group. When feelings, delirious ideas and powerful beliefs are grafted on to these automatisms, it is very difficult for the questioner to obtain dissociations which permit an accurate estimate of the share of the various elements in the hallucinatory complex unless there is an extremely marked predominance. This difficulty is a common clinical observation.

To sum up, it seems that in spite of the absence, in pathological experiments—which are crude and of limited range—of any satisfactory isolation of a syndrome corresponding to the injury of a single kinæsthetic co-ordination centre, there is a verbal relay station for the impressions of articulation; and we may speak —always in the dynamic sense—of autonomous verbal kinæsthetic images, analogous to auditory or visual images, but by no means essential for speech, which depends on the phemic co-ordination centre; in any case we shall no longer talk of pseudo 'motor images' combining sensibility and movement in one paradoxical entity.[1]

[1] Whether there is a co-ordination centre for graphic kinæsthetic evocation we have no means of deciding; its existence seems very probable; in fact, in cases of sensory abnormality, the blind who can write, deaf-mutes using hand-language, verbal kinæsthetic representations which are not articulatory acquire such importance that the practical necessity for a special co-ordination centre arises. Helen Keller has thrown much light on the rôle of such representations, or dynamic agents of kinæsthetic evocation:

"When I was a child," she says, "my inner speech was inner spelling. Although I am even now frequently caught spelling to myself on my fingers, yet I talk to myself, too, with my lips, and it is true that when I first learned to speak, my mind discarded the finger-symbols and began to articulate. However, when I try to rccall what someone has said to me, I am conscious of a hand spelling into mine" (*The World I Live in*, pp. 146-7). For Helen Keller a 'verbal touch' took the place of verbal audition.

8. *Verbal Thought and Wernicke's Aphasia*

Though it is of primary importance for psycho-physiological analysis to throw light on disorders bearing solely, or with a marked predominance, on any special co-ordinative apparatus, this is not so in clinical treatment, for most cases which present themselves are very similar complexes and generally have a very clear pathological significance. In this respect Pierre Marie's classification of aphasias is in complete harmony with current practice. He distinguishes true aphasia, Wernicke's aphasia (Dejerine's sensory aphasia) anarthria (aphemia) which he does not regard as an aphasia, and Broca's aphasia (or Wernicke's aphasia plus anarthria) corresponding to Dejerine's total aphasia.

Aphasia is the common state accompanying right hemiplegia in general, and consists in a lack of comprehension of language in all forms, with no disturbance of elocution, but with paraphasia, or rather jargonophasia, that is to say an incomprehensible verbalism.

In these cases it is the intellectual function of language that is affected, and not sensory reception or motor realization. Though the denial of pure verbal blindness or verbal deafness is not justified, their elimination from the category of aphasia, for the same reason as in the case of aphemia, would certainly be possible, if by definition we were to reserve the term 'aphasia' for disorders of the intellectual function of language.

But what is this function?

In the education of the child, a certain auditory impression acquires significance through the realization of well-known processes which give rise to conditioned reflexes: the word or the phrase arouses the expectation of an agreeable or disagreeable event, with which it has frequently been associated in experience, and so it involves feelings and images—by evocation of the event in question and the circumstances which happen to surround it—and, in particular, appropriate attitudes and reactions. Some of these reactions are verbal—certain vocal manifestations, spontaneous (cries), imitative or learned ("if you please," "excuse me") —which may have an influence on the outcome, favourable or preventive.

With the progress of science, associations (mnemonic evocation, affective impression, adoption of attitudes and preparation for reactions) multiply with a constantly increasing rapidity: as a result of the relations which are established between all experiences they increase in geometrical progression. Except for a few expressions whose signification becomes powerfully automatized, and which are in constant relation with particular events involving the same reaction (the: "Good morning, how do you do?—Quite well thank you and how are you?"), the associations aroused by language are determined by a host of past and present factors (environment, previous conversation, nature of dominant preoccupations, etc.) so that the same word can be understood in very different ways, can, that is to say, arouse quite different feelings, attitudes and mnemonic evocations according to the individual and the occasion.

The functioning of the nervous apparatus which ensures this direction of associations requires not only the integrity of the centre of sensory co-ordination, the importance of which we have shown, but that of the whole group of association circuits which connect this centre with the affective area, with the motor centres and motor co-ordination centres, with all the sensory areas where the concrete mnemonic evocations occur, and finally which connect a given element with various others of the same centre.

This totality of associations which are provoked and which may continue for a long time—each affective, motor or sensory evocation being a starting-point for new associations which enter into competition or are combined—this whole, which constitutes the process of thought, may be realized, especially in cultivated individuals who have enjoyed a well-developed verbal education and experience of words, with a marked predominance in the sphere of language: the evocations aroused by a word may be especially verbal images, which arouse others, and thought will then be concerned almost exclusively with internal speech. It would seem that in the process thought tends to lose its biological characteristic of preparation for more or less differentiated action—the reflex constituting the immediate action—and becomes a self-sufficient process, an end and no longer only a means.[1] Talking to oneself, indeed, is regarded by Pierre Janet as the characteristic feature of psychical activity.[2]

In reality, language, no less than the concrete evocations for which words are often simply substitutes, may constitute an anticipated representation of possible experiences, economizing these experiences, and thus preparing, from a greater distance and in more roundabout ways, the adapted reactions. Nor must it be forgotten that in social life language itself is a form of action, perhaps the most important form in modern civilization, and that internal speech is then no longer an indirect and symbolic representation, but rather a direct representation of experience: the orator thinking of his speech, the professor thinking of his lecture, the writer thinking of his novel, even the philosopher thinking of his theory, are really seeing and preparing in advance their social action. It is possible that this preparation is not followed by the act itself, the complete realization, in speech or writing, but it is none the less

[1] Bergson has made the important suggestion that human thought has freed itself from mere reaction. But the liberation appears especially in reverie and in dream, when there is exhaustion or repose of the higher sensori-motor adaptation.

[2] *Cf.* Pierre Janet, "La tension psychologique, ses dégrés, ses oscillations, II, La hiérarchie des tendances," *British Journal of Psychology*, Medical Section, I, 2, 1921, p. 144.

true that the purpose of the thought was to produce it in a suitable and satisfactory form.

Internal speech, which may serve for the preparation of biological activity, in the struggle with the physical and living environment, is the essential instrument by which we prepare for social activity, in relation to the complex environment constituted by society.

If internal speech can serve for dreams as well as concrete imagination, it is during states of repose, in which the mental functioning is out of order, when the complex of tendencies which constitutes the biological and social personality is relaxed and no longer serves to direct and check with the necessary force. And in this case thought continues to imagine experiences, but without any utilitarian direction, in mere play-activity, in spite of the finalistic view implied by the Freudian theory.

Starting from words and ending in words, internal speech, where it is not complicated by other forms of thought, develops in the cerebral area next to the receptive co-ordination centres; for here can be found pegs corresponding to these words and able to ensure its psychical realization, its affective evocation, through action on a sensory, auditory, kinæsthetic or visual area, with the mental habits which make this or that type of evocation habitually predominate.[1]

Thc multiplicity of the centres of sensory co-ordination enables us to understand that the isolated injury of one of them may allow internal speech to persist, although the auditory centre, which is the first to be trained, is almost always the most troublesome to lose.

But it will be realized that if all the centres of sensory co-ordination were simultaneously lacking,

[1] Usually a rapid evocation, outlined rather than realized. The same is still more true for the concrete evocations. A visual image that is judged to be satisfying is incomplete and singularly false when we wish to realize it completely: directly it ensures suitable evocations, and so *plays its part*, it is, in fact, adequate for thought—though it would not do for drawing.

verbal thought would be deprived of any support and would be impossible.[1]

And even without injury to these centres, or if the injury is further complicated by some disturbance of the network of verbal associations which connects these centres with one another and interconnects the elements of each, and which forms a starting-point for the paths that act on the affective area, or on the concrete evocations, or on the motor areas—if the lines are tangled, verbal thought is thereby rendered impossible; and speech, when it is preserved (in consequence of the motor co-ordination centre remaining intact) becomes incoherent, without direction and without control, except for a few automatisms directly produced by the perception of events, and not requiring roundabout ways of thought.

This is exactly what occurs quite frequently in Wernicke's aphasia, where there is injury to the associative

[1] It may be asked whether, in the absence of an image, thought would be possible; after destruction, for example, of the sensory areas, leaving the co-ordination centres intact or at least sufficiently intact. This question might be answered in the affirmative if there really were in the normal state, as has been affirmed, 'imageless thought.' In fact, during rapid and practical thought which does not delay in artistic play with representations, it is certain that feelings of comprehension, doubt, familiarity, etc., which are correlated with attitudes and reactions provoked by a word or an abstract phrase, may occur without the evocation of any one of the innumerable images that can appear during a realization of the associative irradiation emanating from the abstract concept. Such images, in introspective experiments on the nature of general ideas, are often treated as significant, or as the concepts themselves, whereas in fact they are only an example, and often a very inferior one, of the dynamic power of these concepts. But if feelings precede the complete realization of the associations which tend to become irradiated, they spring from a schematic realization (the feeling of "the word on the tip of the tongue" for example). The complete realization of concrete or verbal sensory evocations is necessary, at least at certain moments, as a guarantee and a control. True *comprehension* always consists in the realization of the evocative dynamic centres, or at least of a certain number of them. The feeling of comprehension at which we generally stop when the evocation is outlined with facility is only an indication, which may be erroneous. It is impossible to think with only the feeling of comprehension, analogous to the feeling of recognition, without either the realization of an act or the awakening of a sensation. Some support is still necessary, a perception or an image, to arouse the feeling; the feelings do not spring up of themselves.

mechanism, the intellectual function of language, as Pierre Marie has well insisted; so that we cannot call this aphasia 'sensory.'[1]

What exactly is the injury to the intelligence in an aphasic patient of the usual type?

If we mean by intelligence a certain quality of mental functioning, vivacity, readiness of adaptation, etc., this quality may be preserved in non-verbal associative functioning, which is all that remains in the case of the uneducated deaf-mute; and in such a case we may say, with Dejerine and Brissot,[2] that the intelligence is not affected, and that there is no demential weakening. But frequently also the cerebral injury involves diffuse manifestations and a general intellectual weakening, which is not at all surprising, though it is not conditioned by the aphasia.[3]

But, if we designate as intelligence, quantitatively, the totality of mental functioning,[4] it is evident that the suppression of verbal thought involves a defect, relatively very important among cultivated individuals leading a complex social life: the uneducated person from this point of view is a defective.

The non-verbal thought of the uneducated deaf-mute

[1] But when the retrocession occurs, there is often a predominance on the side of verbal deafness or verbal blindness. The tracts coming from one of these centres may be severely injured, and there are tracts which remain more affected than others. The lesion does not generally involve a definite and complete destruction.

[2] *Cf.* M. Brissot, *L'aphasie dans ses rapports avec les démences et les vésanies*, 1910.

[3] Forel's auto-observation is very interesting in this connection: he was affected by slight aphasic disorders, with a temporary incapacity to pronounce certain consonants, and it had become impossible for him to make calculations, because of confusions and continual forgetting (*cf. Journal für Psych. und Neur.*, 1915, XXI, p. 434).

[4] From the point of view of measurements and scales of *intelligence*, in applied psychology, the attempt is being made, on the lines laid down by Binet, to furnish numerical support for a judgment of value as to the comparative level of the complex mental functioning of a number of individuals, the resultant of independent and heterogeneous functions; a judgment analogous to one dealing with the beauty of a face as a simultaneous function of the nose, mouth, eyes, complexion, etc.

is, however, biologically a human type of thought, which profits from the broad associative capacities of the brain of man and from an aptitude particularly developed to profit by experience, in proportion as the deaf-mute is not mentally deficient. The imitation of attitudes and gestures also involves a certain social behaviour, though it is only elementary.

The non-verbal thought of the cultivated aphasic patient will perhaps be biologically less rich than that of the deaf-mute, because it may have atrophied in part under the influence of the enormous development of verbal thought; it will be socially more complex on the other hand, because, thanks to language, certain more subtle attitudes and reactions have been learned, which have become automatic or at least freed from language, and which will persist.[1] Feelings and tendencies are refined and extended, and they continue to govern conduct, living their own life even when deprived of the verbal root which was necessary for their original development.

Moreover, the aphasic patient in his mode of life, in his acts and in all his behaviour may seem biologically and socially normal. But he has nevertheless suffered an unquestionable loss, for he no longer has any chance of undergoing further modifications of social origin, and of reacting in his turn as a factor in evolution and progress.

He lacks even the power of using such instruments as are furnished by the social environment and serve both for the stabilization and the development of social relations and for the economy of individual thought with a view to action on the

[1] This difference also remains that when there is a destructive lesion the verbal educability—lacking the appropriate cerebral area—is almost nil, as contrasted with what we find in deaf-mutes. The re-education of aphasic patients is in reality conditioned by incomplete lesions with retrocession — not forgetting the possibility of true substitutions, which are, however, very far from having been demonstrated in such cases.

physical and animate environment; namely, logic, science, etc.[1]

Actions and attitudes persist, governed by feelings and tendencies due to philosophical speculation, scientific research, and moral judgments, either personal or, more probably, derived, but the possibility of again taking up such speculation, research or criticism, or of borrowing from others, is almost altogether lost. Concrete discoveries may still be made; but calculation and especially algebra, which requires symbols, and abstract developments based on concepts implying verbal chains, all become impossible. From verbal education, however, there may remain certain affective irradiations[2] about concrete images and gestures, which have been associated with abstract words (fatherland, love, etc.), and which preserve the meaning and even the use of the concepts expressed by these words.[3] There are, too, non-verbal concepts in the case of the uneducated deaf-mute, and the difference between verbal and non-verbal thought is one of degree of complexity rather than of kind; this complexity is, however, indispensable for the progress of collective instrumenta-

[1] Interesting analyses by Van Woerkom have shown a general incapacity in aphasics for grasping relations, realizing ordered syntheses, etc.; all of them operations which are based, in the normal individual, on the use of verbal symbolization. When confronted by groups of figures or of geometrical forms, the aphasic, even though he may perceive them correctly, is unable to analyse or to order the elements, to grasp their succession or to conceive direction in space ("Sur l'état psychique des aphasiques," *L'Encéphale*, 1923, XVIII, pp. 286-305).

[2] The rôle of affective irradiation in concepts appears with great clearness in the case of a blind deaf-mute like Helen Keller, who thus gives significance to words belonging to visual language, without adequate sensory representation, such as the "green of spring" (*cf.* Helen Keller, op. cit., *The World I Live in*, pp. 124, 129-131).

[3] The concept is, in fact, essentially a capacity for associative evocation; it has a dynamic reality like the image, and is very close to the image. The term 'schema' used by Revault-d'Allonnes, in his interesting psychological analysis of thought (La mécanisme de la pensée. Les schèmes mentaux," *Revue philosophique*, 1920, 9-10, pp. 161-220) is in danger of implying something static, as is already the case with the term 'image'.

tion, the perfecting of logical and scientific machinery and of moral consciousness.

There is, then, in the case of the aphasic patient, an undeniable intellectual deficit, but with the possible preservation of the associative qualities which determine vivacity and intellectual versatility; and this deficit, which affects symbolic thought, bears above all on the social form of thought, without thereby affecting acquired social behaviour, which is governed by feelings and tendencies that are connected with a different cerebral area, as we shall see later.

To sum up, aphasia is due to a lesion—diffuse, more or less complete, and more or less susceptible of retrocession (compressive hæmorrhages re-absorbed without leaving definite lesions) — in the sphere of verbal thought.[1]

In the aphasia known as 'amnesic' there is a diffuse functional disorder, which goes beyond this sphere and involves not so much an injury to the association paths themselves as a deficiency of nervous impulse. If words are not found, if comprehension is slow, and if evocation does not occur readily, it is because the impulse is insufficient to overflow the dams, to overcome the resistances encountered and to affect the neurones with a definite heterochronism; in true aphasia the telephonic lines are mixed and tangled, and there is only cacophony and chaos; in amnesic aphasia, conversation may be rendered impossible because from one station to the other nothing is heard, or only certain easy words, separately, owing to the lack of a sufficient current on the line. The amnesic phenomenon alone is

[1] The co-ordination centres may even be untouched, in which case we may be dealing with echolalia, a psittacistic repetition—without comprehension—of words heard, coexistent with jargonophasia. The direct association of the auditory co-ordination centre with the phemic co-ordination centre—sometimes separately interrupted—is then preserved, in spite of the injury to the associative area of verbal thought. In a case cited by Pfersdorff, there was even, besides repetition without comprehension, automatic elocution lacking sense though correct in form ("Les aphasies transcorticales," Soc. de Médicine du Bas-Rhin, *Presse Médicale*, Feb. 15, 1922, p. 141).

in operation in this last case, a functional disorder of association; in aphasia, there is a specific lesion bearing on the area of the association paths involved in verbal thought.[1]

9. *Head's Attempt at Analysis*

Since aphasia appears as an intellectual disturbance of language, its various degrees, particularly during functional recovery, when, for example, a hæmorrhage is absorbed, follow the hierarchy of the verbal function, and the psycho-pathological data may be usefully compared with linguistic data, such as emerge especially from the important work of Meillet and his pupil Vendryès.[2] Pick had already attempted this in the first part, which is all that has appeared, of his work on the 'Agrammatism'[3] characterized by 'pidgin' language or the 'telegraphic style', a juxtapositon of invariable words, lacking subtleties of form and syntax, and limited to the essential primitive form of 'word-phrases.'

But Head, while he seems to go even further than Pierre Marie—denying sensory or motor aphasias, eliminating anarthria, and seeing in aphasia only an injury to symbolic thought[4]—endeavours to analyse the latter into more elementary functions, which can be isolated, in localized cerebral lesions, as he has already attempted to analyse the functions of sensory thought.

Head is very considerate of the claims of science, as all his work proves, and is not content with clinical schemata, which are all that is necessary for medical

1 But amnesic phenomena through diffuse functional disturbance often complicate aphasic phenomena due to more or less extended lesions of the language area.

2 *Cf.* Vendryès, *Language* (History of Civilization), 1924.

3 Arnold Pick, *Die agrammatischen Sprachstörungen*, I, 1913.

4 In fact, Head eliminates from aphasia the isolated injury of motor expression, verbal apraxia, or the verbal agnosias, whose existence he does not deny; for him such disorders have nothing to do with aphasia; but this seems to be going a little too far.

practice. He submitted aphasic patients during the war to series of tests, affording an opportunity for an analysis of verbal and general behaviour; and this analysis has led him to distinguish four forms of aphasia, which may appear either in an almost pure state, or in combination, with one or other predominating.[1]

To these four forms he gives the names, 'verbal,' 'nominal,' 'syntactical,' and 'semantic' aphasia.

Verbal aphasia is characterized by a defect in the *formation* of words: evocation is difficult, vocabulary limited, and enunciation slow and halting; the same defect occurs in writing. Spelling is defective. There is difficulty in reading, owing to an incapacity to recall a long series of words. Numbers are less affected. When an enunciation is incorrect the patient perceives it. Jokes are well understood whether set out in print or in pictures. Drawing is accurate and also card-playing.

In nominal aphasia it is the *comprehension of the nominal value* of words and symbols in general which is defective, and consequently their use is hampered. Reading is very difficult, spelling and writing are much affected, and copying in freehand is impossible. Complex orders are executed with difficulty. Though numeration is still possible, calculation is no longer so, the significance of numbers being lost. The appreciation of coin-value is defective. The patient can no longer play cards, but can sometimes still play draughts or chess.

Syntactical aphasia is characterized by *jargonophasia*. The articulation and the rhythm of the phrase are defective and grammatical incoherence is complete. Reading is possible, but not verbal formulation. Writing, although less affected, also shows a slight tendency to jargon.

Finally, in semantic aphasia, the *full significance* of

[1] H. Head, "Aphasia and Kindred Disorders of Speech," *Brain*, 1920, XLIII, pp. 87-165; "Disorders of Symbolic Thinking and Expression," *Brit. Journal of Psychology*, 1921, XI. pp. 179-193; "Aphasia: an Historical Review," *Proc. Royal Soc. of Medicine*, 1920, XIV, pp. 1-22.

words and phrases is lost. Separately, each word or each detail of a drawing can be understood, but the general significance escapes; an act is executed upon command, though the purpose of it is not understood. Reading and writing are possible as well as numeration, the correct use of numbers; but the appreciation of arithmetical processes is defective. There is no capacity to play cards correctly, and jokes, written or depicted, are rarely understood. A general conception cannot be formulated, but details can be enumerated.

To sum up: for Head the mental activity of formulation and symbolic expression implies a high degree of integration, and its disturbances cannot be limited to defects of speech, reading, or writing which are not individualized psychic functions. It includes cortical and sub-cortical mechanisms, whose predominance in certain areas of one of the cerebral hemispheres explains the appearance of aphasic disturbances as a result of limited lesions of the brain.

If the lesion specially affects the area of the ascending convolutions we get verbal aphasia: the patient has difficulty in finding the verbal forms necessary for the expression of his thought. If the temporal lobe is particularly affected, the result is jargonophasia and syntactic aphasia. Finally, a lesion situated between the post-central fissure and the occipital lobe disturbs the appreciation of signification: when it is only a matter of verbal signification (nominal aphasia) it is the use of words that is impaired; when the general signification is more disturbed (semantic aphasia) the comprehension of logical conceptions is lacking.[1]

Head's attempt at analysis is very interesting, and the isolation of functions, which might be separately

[1] *Cf.* Henry Head, "Speech and Cerebral Localization," *Brain*, 1923, XLVI, pp. 355-528. In this fine study we have a very full account of five highly characteristic observations, dealing with cerebral lesions. The localizations in the different cases discussed are not based on anatomical examinations, *post mortem*, but on what could be ascertained as to the injuries of the living patient.

abolished, according to the seat of the lesion, would be of great importance. Unfortunately the types of disorder are still insufficiently clear and seem to be very complex. They are groups of disturbances presenting such considerable individual differences that we are tempted to suppose that the four functions are either too many or too few.

The last type is related to a very diffuse intellectual disturbance, a weakening of the most complex associative functions. The first two would imply a predominance either in expression or in comprehension, and are, in short, very like the old types of aphasia with a motor or sensory predominance. The jargonophasic type—which is often associated with others—evidently involves a disorder which attracts attention and enables it to be individualized; it would be essentially the equivalent of 'agrammatism.'

What, in any case, particularly emerges from this whole group of studies is the relation of an injury to a limited temporo-parieto-occipital area, in the left brain, with disturbances of nominal or semantic comprehension, that is to say with the most characteristic disturbance of symbolic thought, which in man, the speaker, is essentially verbal thought.

Experiments on aphasics open the way to a finer analysis—psychological and cerebrological—of symbolic thought, thanks to the initiative of Head, the value of which cannot be too strongly emphasized.[1]

[1] The capital importance of the researches of Head has been very rightly noted by H. Delacroix in his remarkable book, *Le Langage* (Paris, 1924).

Chapter III

THE PROBLEM OF VERBAL LOCALIZATION AND APHASIA

It is a very widespread opinion, but one which is none the less entirely inaccurate, that none of the cerebral localizations relative to language can be maintained to-day. Though different views are opposed to the old ones, there are unquestionable anatomo-pathological facts in evidence of localization, which, though less exact than we might wish, is much more so than certain writers would have us believe.

To begin with, we know that in the great majority of cases, the lesions which involve disorders of speech and language are those of the left hemisphere, and injuries to the left brain during the war have once more fully demonstrated this. Moreover, aphasia is most often accompanied by right hemiplegia. There are, however, individual differences, and there are people who from the point of view of language are cerebrally right-handed; and it has frequently been observed that left-handed people, whose motor predominance is governed by the right hemisphere, and who are consequently cerebrally right-handed for movements of the hand, are also cerebrally right-handed for language.

But the connection is not necessary, and cases have been observed, though in very rare exceptions, where aphasia was produced by a lesion of the right hemisphere among right-handed people, with a motor predominance of the left hemisphere, or indeed where aphasia was produced by the lesion of the left hemisphere among left-handed people.[1]

In any case the function of language is connected asymmetrically with the integrity of one of the cerebral hemispheres alone, and that of itself implies a localization.

In the second place, it can be stated that aphemia on the one hand, and Wernicke's aphasia on the other, as Pierre Marie also maintained, are conditioned by lesions

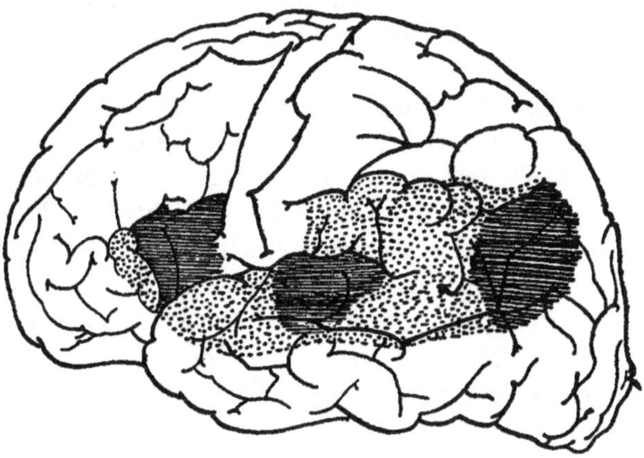

FIG. 17. The centres of language according to the classic conception (Dejerine).

In front, the dark area represents Broca's centre or the centre of motor images of words, the lesion of which involves aphemia (foot of the third frontal); in the middle, above the first temporal, the centre of auditory images of words, the lesion of which involves verbal deafness; and behind, at the level of the angular gyrus, the centre of visual images of words, the lesion of which involves verbal blindness. All the dotted temporo-parietal region is Wernicke's area.

of totally different regions of the hemisphere concerned. Comparison of the clinical data has established the fact that, in the first case, the lesion is located in the large cerebral quadrilateral known as the lenticular area, which includes cortical elements (the insula) and subcortical elements (internal capsular fibres, the lenticular

[1] *Cf.* K. Mendel, "Ueber Rechtshirnigkeit bei Rechthändern," *Neurol. Centralblatt*, XXXIII, 5, p. 291; Long, "Un case d'aphasie par lésion de l'hémisphère gauche chez un gaucher," *L'Encéphale*, 1913, pp. 520-536.

nucleus of the striate body, and the claustrum); in the second case, the lesion extends throughout Wernicke's zone at the confluence of the three lobes, temporal, parietal and occipital.

The legend of the failure of localization follows quite simply—if we free the anatomical problem from psychological theories—from the fact that Broca's centre, the foot of the third frontal, considered as the seat of the lesion peculiar to aphemia, has become discredited and is eliminated from Pierre Marie's quadrilateral, which stops at this point.

But whether the lesion of aphemia should be exactly at the foot of the third frontal or a little farther on—the errors of the various authors being explained by the frequency of the concomitant degeneration of Broca's area from arterial embolism which, in the neighbourhood of the fissure of Sylvius, usually causes aphasia—hardly affects the notion of localization. As a matter of fact, Pierre Marie is not very definite, for, like a wise clinician, he objects to theoretical constructions and premature hypotheses.

Although a tentative theory of aphemia—designated by the term 'anarthria'—as a simple difficulty of articulation, has doubtless seemed compatible with injuries of the sub-cortical centres, such as the lenticular nucleus (though such a theory has never been expressly formulated), what appears to be essential in the large quadrilateral is the region of the insula, which in a sense forms the prolongation of the base of the third frontal, without any precise limitation, together with individual variations for the division of the architectonic areas.[1]

And, though we can no longer admit that aphemia results from the loss of motor images of words, deposited

1 The insula and Broca's centre surround the Rolandic opercula where are located the incito-motor labio-glosso-laryngeal elements, with bilateral action, the injury of which gives us a picture of pseudo-bulbar paralysis, with dysarthria but without aphemia.

in the cells of the cortex, but must suppose that elocution depends on a motor co-ordination centre, we are justified in localizing this centre in the region of the

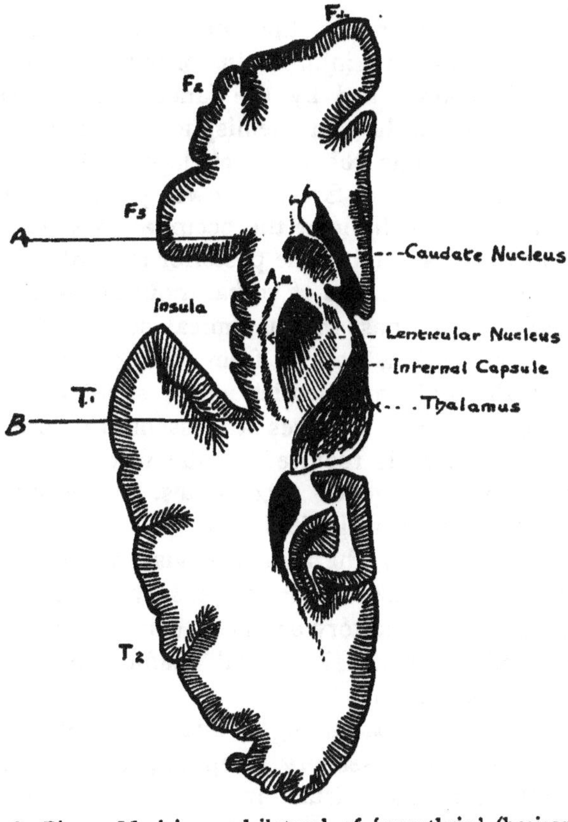

FIG. 18. Pierre Marie's quadrilateral of 'anarthria' (horizontal section of the brain).

The area between the two lines A and B, including the Insula between the edges of the fissure of Sylvius, the anterior wall (A. *w*) the striate body (lenticular nucleus and caudate nucleus), the thalamus, and the extremities of the external and internal capsules, but leaving out the third frontal (F 3), and the temporals, which form part of Wernicke's zone below the quadrilateral.

insula, in the immediate neighbourhood of Broca's centre and perhaps impinging more or less on it. In any case, there is a cerebral area in the anterior part of one hemisphere, nearly always the left, the exact limits of which are not established, but whose integrity is necessary to elocution, regarded as an independent function.

On the other hand, the intellectual function of language which is injured in ordinary Wernicke's aphasia is conditioned by the functional integrity of a cerebral area in the same hemisphere, situated further back and including the area enveloping the posterior part of the fissure of Sylvius (lower parietal convolution as far as the limit of the occipital, first temporal and part of the second in the posterior region).

Here we have the area of verbal thought: so that this form of thought has an anatomical seat, and Pierre Marie's conception, so far from being the weapon against all localizing theories which some have tried to make it, rather involves an essentially localizing principle such as is required by the facts themselves, since verbal intelligence necessitates, in his opinion, the integrity of a very limited area.

But, on this view, the area is envisaged as a single whole, with no dissociation of sensory verbal centres which condition auditory or visual comprehension and are injured separately in verbal deafness and verbal blindness respectively.

The area of verbal thought would lie between the common centres of sensory reception, auditory in the temporal area and visual in the occipital, though without including them.

But, as we have seen, there are cases of pure verbal blindness of which the war lesions provided further examples, as Pierre Marie has recognized,[1] and even cases of pure verbal deafness. Here the lesions are

[1] Pierre Marie's explanation, as given by Chatelin, shows by its lack of precision the difficulty of making the newly recognized facts agree with the earlier negative theory: "It is the combination of a lesion of the visual area with comparatively slight damage to this zone of language, or the fibres proceeding from it, which constitutes alexia." *Les blessures du cerveau*, p. 140. E.T., p. 136.

different and are found at the opposite limits of Wernicke's zone : in verbal blindness they are located either in the cortex or in the white matter, at the limits of the occipital lobe towards the region of the angular gyrus ; in verbal deafness, in the middle of the temporal area.

Limited areas, therefore, certainly exist in the sphere of verbal thought, corresponding to centres of sensory co-ordination the existence[1] of which is required both by clinical facts and by psycho-physiological analysis.

It is impossible to determine precisely the limits of these centres. Does the angular gyrus which was regarded as the seat of visual images of words (and which might be the relay station ensuring the dynamic co-ordination whereby images are produced, but which probably plays a rôle especially in the co-ordination of motor reflexes of visual origin) really correspond to this function, as Dejerine would have us believe? It is still impossible to give a definite answer. But it is perhaps in the occipital lobe itself, on the lower internal surface, or perhaps in the angular gyrus,[2] in any case fairly close to it, that we should look for the centre of visual co-ordination implied both by rapid reading and by the evocation of verbal visual repre-

[1] In Henschen's fine publications, co-ordinating the results of 700 anatomo-pathological observations of aphasia, we find clear indications of definite localization, different for language, music and calculation, and even partial localizations and words and syllables. Though the general conceptions of Henschen, who adheres to classic doctrines, can no longer be accepted, the facts, which ought to be incorporated in the new interpretations, cannot be neglected (*cf.* S. E. Henschen, *Klinische und anatomische Beiträge zur Pathologie des Gehirns*, Henschen's own summaries ("Les altérations de la faculté du langage, de la musique et du calcul" *Rev. Neurol* 1920, XXVII pp. 1089-1094) and those of André Thomas ("Aphasie, amusie, et acalculie d'après Henschen," *L'Encéphale*, December, 1921, pp. 605-614).

[2] The lesion of the white matter which interrupts the left optic radiations and involves verbal blindness is included between the angular gyrus on the external surface of the hemisphere and the cuneus or the lingual lobe on its internal surface. Chatelin inclines to place the lesion conditioning alexia in the fusiform lobe or the lingual lobe. It is, of course possible that the interruption of the tracts of access to the co-ordination centre may be mistaken for a lesion of the centre itself: many association tracts of the optic area pass near the angular gyrus.

sentations (hence the inexactitude of the term alexia, which Pierre Marie and his pupils prefer for theoretical reasons).

The centre of auditory co-ordination for the comprehension of speech and the evocation of auditory representations is located in the temporal lobe, though we can neither delimit it very precisely nor determine its relations to the auditory receptive area, about which, unlike the occipital visual area, relatively little is known.

As for the probable centre of kinæsthetic co-ordination, which may be placed between the temporal auditory centre and the motor area, the absence of sufficiently clear clinical data does not as yet allow localization, in the proper sense of the word.

Aphemia, like apraxia, is connected with an injury to the mechanism of motor co-ordination, and this mechanism has a cerebral seat which we can place almost exactly. The centre of graphic co-ordination where the lesion of agraphia is located is situated at the edge of the base of the second frontal and the ascending frontal, at the level of the incito-motor centres for the hand.

The other forms of apraxia depend on analogous but less complex mechanisms, the seat of which we have not yet been able to determine with certainty, or even approximately; we only know that it must also be sought as a rule in the left hemisphere, and that it may be found neither in the occipital area nor in the temporal but only in the fronto-parietal. Vague though it still is, this first approximate localization is already a considerable achievement.

Similarly agnosias, losses of perceptive comprehension for common objects are connected with lesions of one hemisphere only, nearly always the left: though occipital lesions give hemianopsias, right or left according to the hemisphere damaged, we still sometimes find visual agnosias with right hemianopsias, in spite of the preservation of macular vision, as we have already pointed out. Verbal blindness itself, a more limited agnosia, coincides nearly always with this same right hemianopsia. A lesion which involves functional loss of the mechanism of verbal visual co-ordination may, in fact, extend to the occipital area of direct reception, or especially affect the radiations which bring the visual impulses to this occipital area, radiations which pass under Wernicke's zone and enter this area in the infra-structure of the angular gyrus.

We know enough then to assume, on anatomical grounds and without any imaginary constructions, the existence of limited cerebral areas corresponding to the sensory or motor co-ordinating functions implied by psycho-physiological analysis—the existence, that is to say, of real *co-ordination centres.*

We also know enough to affirm that round the co-ordination centres of verbal reception there extends an associative area[1] which conditions verbal thought. The co-ordination centres are the points of insertion through which sensory impressions act and from which concrete evocations start; they are the supports without which the entire structure crumbles, and all verbal functioning becomes impossible; but this functioning cannot continue, even though the co-ordination centres remain intact, if the association paths get confounded by a lesion that injures the area of verbal thought as a whole.

So long as the associations which arise from the other sensory impressions, feelings, attitudes, etc., remain possible, non-verbal thought, which is conditioned by

[1] In this area are located numerous cortical relay neurones which serve as points of re-direction, but do not correspond to mental individualizations, which appertain to the excitation of the neurones of the sensory area alone. We cannot regard this as the seat of entities, schemata, or concepts, which are only dynamisms with a sensory support. We may, however, wonder whether the feelings which accompany cerebral functioning do not involve the excitation of certain of these neurones, or whether they are localized in an independent area.

the other association paths as a whole—with peculiar forms linked also to limited areas[1]—may continue normally, if functional disorders, resulting from the pathological accident which produced the aphasia, do not extend to the entire brain.

And the progress of our knowledge of nervous functioning allows us to conceive of the part played by the relay stations throughout this dynamic mental system, by that neuronic syntonization whose mechanism we outlined above (see Chap. V. of Part II.).

In reality, our anatomo-physiological conception of language and thought is gradually improving, gaining in exactness what it may lose in apparent precision. We must renounce—as previously for the re-direction of neurones by amœbism—the idea of three or four reservoirs of images, painted in blue or red on diagrams of the brain, but this does not mean that we must renounce the localization of the real functions which have taken the place of the entities with which the localizers of earlier times worked.

It need not greatly surprise us that our attention to scientific exactitude does not give us more precision, for some of the chief reasons can readily be indicated:

To begin with, we find ourselves dealing with rough and generally diffuse injuries, in extraordinarily complex and delicate mechanisms, involving complex clinical states; we cannot experiment, and it is to the unhappy accidents of pathology alone that we owe the possibility of extending our knowledge of the lesional processes due to vascular disorders (embolism and hæmorrhage), which depend on the distribution of the arteries and do not oblige us by limiting themselves to small areas with autonomous functions. The wounds and injuries caused by projectiles during the war—generally also complicated by hæmorrhages and vascular disturbances

[1] Thus thought, by visual schematization, depends particularly on the association paths near the occipital lobe, and orientation alone may be injured in certain limited lesions, etc.

—the microscopic overflow due to concussion, gave rise to disturbances less ordinary though sufficiently complex. But in only a few cases could anatomical examination complete the clinical analyses.

Again, functional analysis generally remains very rudimentary and limited to the needs of the clinic; while the great majority of the available anatomical examinations are also very inadequate. Localizations have been established according to the morphology of the convolutions, which have no necessary connection with the functional areas: they correspond to the cell structures which the cyto-architectonic of the brain has begun to establish, and which often cover different convolutions.

Another new difficulty lies in the individual variability which is possible in psycho-physical mechanisms, and which is beyond doubt constitutional: cerebrally right- and left-handed individuals provide an obvious example of this. The cyto-architectonic shows that the relations of functional areas with a morphological appearance vary greatly with the individual, so that any judgment based on the appearance of the convolutions—which are already so variable—is suspect. Finally Moutier has emphasized the extraordinary variability of arterial distribution, of the vascular divisions and channels, in particular in the area of the fissure of Sylvius, which results in great differences in the complexity of lesions for an arterial embolus of a given trunk, according to the topographical type.

Add to this the great difficulty that we feel—especially when we have not been able to follow their evolution for long—in distinguishing disorders due to a true, irremediable, irreversible destruction, from functional ones, due to distant causes and sometimes lasting, which, when the retrocession occurs, prevent our assigning limits to the anatomical area that corresponds to them (a metabolism more or less affected by insufficient irrigation, compression, inflammation, etc.), to say nothing of the reverberations of diaschisis in the partially affected circuits.[1]

Finally, considerable difficulties of interpretation are involved by the functional equivalence of the complete isolation of a centre through interruption of all its association paths and the destruction of this centre itself, separately, as contrasted with the very great difference in the appearance of lesions which are limited to the white matter in the one case and may be more or less limited to the grey matter of the cortex in the other. Interminable discussion may arise, for example, as to the significance of the angular gyrus in verbal blindness or of the base of the second frontal in agraphia, not to mention the fact that a complete or partial interruption of a great association bundle with a determined function (occipito-frontal, occipito-temporal, etc.), can occur at very different points of its extent with like results.

There even appears to be the possibility, in certain cases, though obviously much more rarely than is supposed, of functional recovery through the substitution (of one hemispere for the other, for example, in praxic or gnosic co-ordination) of other cerebral areas, where a given functional area may be reconstituted.

Considering our difficulties, then, it is no mean achievement to have succeeded in limiting, even if somewhat vaguely, the areas in which certain centres are found or through which great association paths

[1] This difficulty, even with a satisfactory correlation of psycho-physiological and cyto-architectonic examinations, will long preclude absolutely precise localization. Moreover this will probably vary too greatly from one individual to another, and involves groups of keys on the co-ordinative keyboard of language. But the existence of such localizations admits of no doubt when, with minimal lesions, we find limited disturbances not following Ribot's law of regression relative to the disappearance of mechanisms in an inverse order from their automatization. In diffuse and incomplete functional injury this law is essentially valid; and I found a very good example in one of my cases, where aphasia resulted from an insufficient irrigation of the anterior and middle left brain, as the result of a ligature of the primary carotid. Henschen's evidence, too, provides some very clear anatomo-pathological cases of dissociation, showing isolated injuries of the co-ordinative keys.

pass, such as those which condition verbal thought. And we must not expect rapid progress.[1] But the essentials are certainly there, and that suffices to provide a general conception, until more detailed investigation leads to more satisfactory results. There is an unquestionable correspondence between determined functions and definite cerebral areas, and though the localizations may at one time have seemed more precise they have never been more firmly grounded. This conclusion is inevitable for all who are acquainted with the facts and are honest with themselves.

[1] It must not be forgotten that even for the elementary functions, which lend themselves to direct experimentation, there are reflex centres which are not yet precisely localized. The centres of muscular tonus in mammals are still determined only hypothetically. A fortiori, when we come to human reflexes, the uncertainty is even more remarkable. Not only are certain co-ordination centres for ocular movements still unknown, but even the patellar reflex has been located in the brain or in the lower spinal segments; those of the cutaneous reflexes in the cerebral cortex or in the lower part of the spinal cord. And if war pathology has furnished data which are in many cases decisive, it is not less true that such uncertainty as to the seat of the reflex connecting neurones which govern the most simple reactions, and whose existence is unquestionable, shows us how cautious we must be when we encounter uncertainties or contradictions as to the localization of the connecting neurones involved in extraordinarily complex functions.

PART IV

THE AFFECTIVE REGULATION OF MENTAL LIFE
ITS RÔLE AND MECHANISM

CHAPTER I

THE IDEA OF LIBERATION OF ENERGY AND 'INTEREST'

THE study of the cerebral associative mechanisms on which the processes of perception and the forms of thought depend does not exhaust the problem of mental activity.

The dynamic standpoint of evolutionary biology, which dominates contemporary psychology, demands that we should occupy ourselves with the actual operation of these mechanisms. When we consider mental functioning in action, even assuming that we know all the groups of neurones implicated in a given process, we still have to determine what causes this process, and on what energy it draws. There is a quantitative aspect in mental action seen as a whole, with which the remarkable work of Pierre Janet is connected. And this quantitative aspect involves complicated distinctions.[1]

Mental activity is a function of an expenditure of nervous energy, each neurone furnishing, as it consumes

[1] F. H. Pike has observed that the introduction of the idea of changes in the quantity of nervous energy (Hughlings Jackson) for given systems of afferent pathways as a result of partial lesions, might allow us to determine cerebral localization more exactly than did Monakow ("Remarks on von Monakow's *Die Lokalisation im Grosshirn*," *Journal of Comparative Neurology*, 1918, XXIX, 5, pp. 485-508).

cell reserves, a process of excitation capable of stimulating, in other neurones, expenditures of their own which in their turn require a new using up of reserves. Whether the reserves are exhausted, as in the last stages of inanition, when the nervous elements can no longer borrow from the other tissues of the organism and when coma sets in; or whether the chemical production of nervous energy is suddenly rendered impossible, through a stoppage of the circulation or a suppression of oxygen, etc., which involves the immediate disappearance of the cerebral functions, the highest showing themselves to be the most delicate: in both cases, mental functioning is abolished through a lack of the necessary energy.

If there is a slight deficiency in the energic processes only the most costly mental activities become impossible, the complex synthetic functions, constructive thought and efforts of attention, while the automatisms continue to work correctly, in states of fatigue, decreased oxygenation, partial anæmia, etc.

But in the absence of any apparent organic cause of modification in nervous metabolism, considerable variations in the level of mental activity and of conduct may be noticed, and these have been systematically analysed by Pierre Janet.[1] Difficult actions requiring considerable expenditure of energy will be possible at some moments and impossible at others.[2] This is perhaps

[1] The notion of levels of activity might be applied to the functioning of the nervous centres, and even in these there would be a level of high tension, according to Head, who has suggested the term 'vigilance' for this higher level of activity at whatever stage it appears. Vigilance thus merges into the higher degrees of attention and mental efficiency in the psychological processes characteristic of the higher stages of the nervous system. *Cf.* H. Head, "Release of Function in the Nervous System," *Proc. Royal Soc.*, 1921, B 92, pp. 184-209—"The conception of Mental and Nervous Energy (Vigilance; a Physiological State of the Nervous System), *VII* (*Oxford*) *International Congress of Psychology, Proceedings and Papers*, Cambridge, 1924, pp. 163-184.

[2] Under the influence of an emotion, the movements of a monkey deprived of the cortical incito-motor centres are more easily carried out (Minkowski). Parkinsonians suffering from mutism, when they are moved, begin to talk

connected, in certain cases, with the existence of reserves of energy which are not renewed and are finally exhausted. But as a rule, and in a constant fashion for normal individuals, the difference will result from the fact that there is a liberation of energy at a given moment which either does not occur at all or occurs at a greatly reduced rate at other moments. In one case, there is a state of thought-relaxation leading to somnolence or to sleep, diffuse thought at the mercy of the haphazard action of associative automatisms and external stimulation—a contracting of mental activity; in the other case, there is a tense condition of attention, the thought being increased and applied to a definite object, so that it can be the source of useful evocations, in virtue of some 'interest,' by which energy is liberated.

What we call 'interest' is this very phenomenon of the liberation of nervous energy, which shows itself as much in the domain of physical activity—up to the point of exhaustion in a runner anxious to beat a speed or endurance record—as in that of mental activity—up to the point of extreme cerebral fatigue in a creative worker in the midst of some lengthy and arduous production.

Interest is the manifestation of the intervention of affective phenomena and tendencies, and varies as one or other of these tendencies predominates. An action may arouse in me a keen interest, but this will suddenly disappear when the uneasiness of expectation polarizes all my mental activity towards the passing moment.

In particular, the liberation of energy—realized under a nervous influence which should be regarded as very similar to trophic influences—though capable of general variations, from the high levels of pleasant excitation

correctly, while voluntary effort, except in verbal reflex reactions, fails to attain anything, insufficient energy being liberated to overcome resistance, especially when this energy is dispersed in the course of an effort of thought (*cf.* Babinski, Jarkowski and Plichet, "Kinésie paradoxale, mutisme parkinsonien," *Revue Neurologique*, 1921, No. 12, pp. 1266-1270.)

to the low degrees of depressive grief, is unequally canalized in many directions.

We cannot imagine mental functioning as the outcome of the passive operation of association chains more or less modified by external stimuli, or by the results of certain motor reactions to which they give rise. This functioning is that of an organism with a reactive power of its own, which appears in what we call the tendencies. The associative instrument is utilized for the needs of a life which obeys congenital impulses, directed by deep affective impressions. Thought provides means of action which may appear as secondary ends; nevertheless, the true ends of action arise not from the neo-mental intellectual area but from the affective or paleo-mental area, which is biologically more primitive, and should be sharply distinguished from it.

CHAPTER II

AFFECTIVE REGULATION IN BIOLOGY

IN the simplest known organisms that have not evolved in the vegetal direction, we find positive or negative reactions in face of external excitations, and it might be supposed that if these excitations suited the interest of the living being, this would be the chance outcome of repeated selection. But we find an aptitude for profiting by experience, the formation, for example, of a negative reaction in the presence of nocuous stimuli, just as if the production of a disagreeable affective impression had involved the reversal of an initial reflex attitude.

Infusoria which ingest grains of carmine with their alimentary particles, soon come to refuse them.

And the fact is still more clearly emphasized when we are dealing with more complicated organisms.[1] An ant which leaps down from a platform where it has been imprisoned, in order to regain its nest, will definitely refuse to do so if once it has fallen into vinegar (Van der Heyde). A lizard which has bitten a worm of offensive odour refuses thenceforward to touch similar worms.

On the other hand, other experiences—which may accordingly be qualified as agreeable—arouse in the future a positive interest, an endeavour to repeat them.

Behaviour is found to be governed by general

[1] See H. Piéron, *L'Évolution de la Mémoire*, Bibl. de Philos scientifique, Paris, 1910.

tendencies whence is derived adaptation to circumstances and to different sorts of environment. The hereditary equipment of reflexes and of instincts—those complicated reflexes which Rabaud often succeeded in separating into their more simple constituents[1]—undergoes, thanks to the play of these affective tendencies, modifications which many facts prove to be hereditarily transmissible, in spite of statements to the contrary which are the outcome of faith in fashionable doctrines.

The mechanism of modification rests in the first place upon a "physiological selection of actions" by the method of trial and error in Jennings' sense.

At a certain stage of evolution, an associative registration of the experience occurs, allowing the appearance of what Yerkes calls "ideative behaviour": and since these experiences may be evoked without being realized, there may be an economy of trial and groping. Intelligence then manifests itself as a "technique of attempts at reaction," to use Claparède's expression. By means of the intellect as an instrument, it substitutes for elementary anticipation, by an associative transference, which seems to be the primitive form of adaptation, a representative adaptation,[2] true prevision.

Reasoning, the most perfect technical form of this kind of process, consists essentially in foreseeing a result and thus doing without some experience whose beginning and end we reconstitute on the basis of what we have already acquired.

But the intellectual instrument, with its mechanical automatisms and its own elaborations, accomplishes the aims of an activity directed by the tendencies, and

[1] See E. Rabaud, *Éléments de Biologie générale*, Paris, 1921.

[2] In this adaptation we have a true conditioned reflex, described in invertebrates even before Pavlov had examined it physiologically and studied it in mammals. I myself described some very clear cases in actinians (*cf.* H. Piéron, "L'étude expérimentale de l'anticipation adaptive," *Association française pour l'Avancement des Sciences. Congrès de Lille*, 1909, pp. 735-739).

cannot, therefore, be considered exhaustively apart from them. The merit of psycho-analysis has been that it has emphasized the rôle of affective factors in the association of ideas, and in the operation of mnemonic processes.

The way in which feelings and tendencies enter into the processes of attention, and even into all logical processes, has been subjected to a most interesting analysis by Rignano.[1] In Ribot's 'affective logic' the rôle of the feelings is evident, but all logic has an affective character, for though one piece of reasoning may, taken in isolation, correspond to an intellectual automatism by conforming to a general model, an acquired social technique, a succession of reasonings—that is to say, a genuine thought process—is always governed by tendencies which have their intellectual counterpart in what are called 'judgments of value,' which are at the beginning of all activity.

Affective processes and associative processes are closely intermingled, and, in the higher emotions, very complex intellectual data mingle with affective impressions; the tendencies subdivide and multiply as functions of a richer and richer experience, which is all the richer because over and above the congenital equipment of instincts and his own personal acquisitions, civilized man receives by education a résumé of social experience individually acquired but of collective origin.

However complicated they may be for psychological analysis, the tendencies are connected at their primary biological foundation with appetition and aversion, which form the greatest obstacles to a mechanistic explanation of life, and which give the vitalists an opportunity of begging the question by making an appeal to a very convenient entity.[2]

[1] Rignano, *The Psychology of Reasoning*, 1923 (in the International Library of Psychology).

[2] *Cf.* H. Piéron, "Du rôle et de la signification du conflit scientifique entre mécanisme et vitalisme," *Scientia*, 1922, pp. 115-126.

In any case, whether or not we seek to explain them by reducing them to something else, the directive tendencies of activity and of organic behaviour are data which cannot be neglected in the study of mental functioning.

Chapter III

THE PHYSIOLOGY OF THE AFFECTIVE LIFE

A 'spinal' mammal, that is to say a mammal subject only to the control of the spinal centres, has no spontaneity; it exhibits reflex mechanisms which may be somewhat complicated, but its activity is governed entirely by external stimuli.

On the other hand, a dog or a cat, even when entirely deprived of the association area, the cerebral cortex, will, if the functions of the paleo-encephalon, and in particular the thalamus, remain intact, behave in a co-ordinated manner; like an individual obedient to tendencies. Thus Dusser de Barenne's decerebrate cat walked about spontaneously, was successful, although blind, in avoiding obstacles, could even, so long as it possessed its olfactory lobes, seek out, find and take its food—without of course being able to capture it—lay down on a rug near the stove, refused absolutely to eat meat soaked with quinine (like the decerebrate dog of Zeliony),[1] and reacted to painful stimuli by threats, mews and growls of anger, and by flight, like the decerebrate monkeys of Karplus and Kreidl, crying out from pain.[2] An anencephalic child makes the same grimaces, when given a bitter solution to taste, as does a normal new-born baby.[3]

[1] G. P. Zeliony, "Observations sur des chiens auxquels on a enlevé les hemispheres cérébraux," *C. R. Soc. de Biologie*, 1913, p. 707.

[2] J. P. Karplus and A. Kreidl, "Ueber Total extirpationen einer und beider Grosshirnhemisphären an Affen (*Macacus rhesus*)," *Archiv. für Physiologie*, 1914, pp. 155-212.

[3] *Cf.* W. Sternberg, "Geschmacksempfindung eines Anencephalus," *Zeitschr. fur Psychologie*, 1901, XXVII, p. 77.

Though the 'thalamic' animal lacks the capacity of appropriate reaction, the delicate perception of events, the plastic adaptation of response and the appeal to memories of earlier experiences, it has still the general direction of an activity which seeks agreeable impressions and tries to avoid painful impressions.

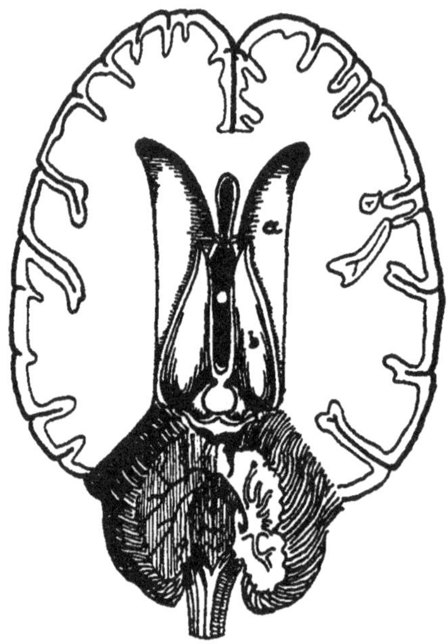

FIG. 19. Horizontal section of the brain (Debierre) showing the 'basal nuclei,' the caudate nucleus (*a*) of the striate body and the optic thalamus (*b*).

Moreover, Goltz even attributed to his decerebrate dog hate, attachment and the maternal and sexual instincts.

In the higher vertebrates, the sphere of affective regulation, the paleo-mental area, is localized in the centres at the base of the brain, in the paleo-encephalon, while the associative intellectual, or neo-mental, area, has its seat in the centres of the cerebral cortex, in the neo-encephalon.

These data are in full agreement with Head's[1] general distinctions, outlined above, according to which sensory excitations produce at the level of the cortex delicate and differentiated perceptive reactions, and at the level of the thalamus, unqualified affective reactions.

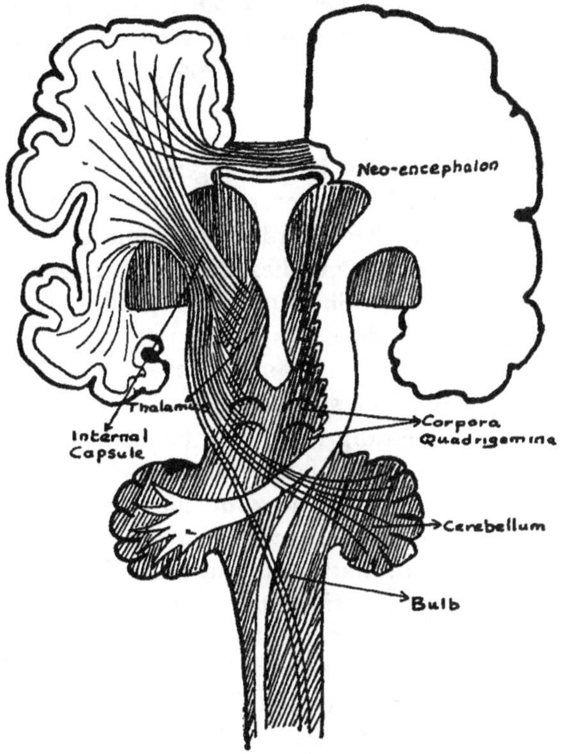

FIG. 20. The paleo-encephalon (in grey) and the neo-encephalon (in white) with its own paths of conduction which have marked out a way in the basal ganglia (after Edinger). The grey ovoid surface traversed by the internal capsule represents the section of the striate body.

The 'interoceptive' sensations, that is to say coenæsthetic impressions give rise especially to affective reactions — which in their turn have an associative

[1] A very general summary of Head's views will be found in his Croonian Lecture of 5th May 1921 (*Proc. Royal Soc.*, 1921, B. 92, No. 645, pp. 184-209).

reverberation and become the object of intellectual experience—unlike the senses specialized for knowledge of the external world, such as sight, which only have a greatly reduced immediate affective reactivity, smell taking an intermediate position.

The rôle of the thalamus in emotional expression and in affective mimicry has long been known. But it has been regarded only as a centre of expressive co-ordination usually acting under the influence of cortical stimulation (Bechterew).

An emotion arising in the higher mental sphere would be translated by appropriate gestures and attitudes, through the key-board of thalamic expression. And when he finds manifestations of anger in a decerebrate animal, Sherrington regards them as "pseudo-affective reflexes." There would be a reflex response released by the same mechanism as in the case of any reflex of the spinal dog.[1]

When, by stimulating not the thalamus itself but the adjacent ganglion, the caudate nucleus which belongs to the striate body, the floor of the fore-brain, the telencephalon of which the cortex is the roof, Pagano obtains all the manifestations of anger or of fear according to the seat of the excitation,[2] the objection is raised that the existence of affective reactions does not prove that the seat of the phenomena of emotion is sub-cortical. If the same reactions are obtained in the case of an animal deprived of its cortex (Pagano), this is taken as a proof that they are pseudo-affective in character;

[1] *Cf.* Sherrington, *The Integrative Action of the Nervous System*, 1906. On the other hand Graham Brown, from his experiments on the emotional mimicries obtained by excitation of the caudal area of the thalamus, concludes only that this area is connected with activities which condition the expressive reactions ("Note on the Physiology of the Basal Ganglia," *Journal of Physiology*, 1915, XLIX, pp. 195-207).

[2] By electrical stimulation of the caudate nucleus (in the thick frontal area of the head) by means of needles previously adjusted, Pachon and Delmas-Marsalet elicited, in two dogs, expressions of satisfaction accompanied by licking ("Effets produits par l'excitation électrique des noyaux caudés chez le chien eveillé," *C. R. Soc. de Biologie*. 1924, XCI, pp. 558-560).

if not (Gemelli), this is said to prove that affective phenomena have a cortical seat, secondary to the subcortical excitation.

We have here the same discussion as arose when Sherrington showed that an 'apesthetized' dog, that is to say a dog deprived, by section of the spinal cord and certain cranial nerves, of all relations between the brain and the viscera, exhibited the same emotions and the same affective reactions as a normal dog. Advocates of a peripheral theory of the emotions, of the Lange type, object that Sherrington's dogs had still the automatic mimicry of affectivity, but no longer felt emotions.

This objection was raised with better justification against the affective manifestations obtained by excitation of the caudate nucleus in apesthetized dogs (Gemelli).[1]

But if we proceed on the subjective ground of an animal's conscious impressions, when we cannot even say for certain whether it is capable of consciousness at all, the discussion is as vain as it is interminable.

The facts show that thalamic activity suffices to govern the general behaviour of an organism, as a function of certain tendencies, with affective regulation, and that thus the automatic reactions of fear, anger and satisfaction take their place in a complex which has real affective value.[2]

[1] See especially on this question: C. S. Sherrington, "Experiment on the Value of Vascular and Visceral Factors for the Genesis of Emotion," *Proc. Royal Soc.* 1900, LXVI, pp. 390-403.—G. Pagano, "Il meccanismo fisiologico dei emozioni," *Riv. di Patol. nerv. e ment.*, 1912, XVII, pp. 687-696.—A. Gemelli, *La teoria somatica dell' Emozione*, 1910.—H. Piéron, "La théorie des émotions et les données actuelles de la physiologie," *Journal de Psychologie*, 1907, IV, pp. 439-451.—G. Dumas, "L'expression des émotions," *Revue Philosophique*, 1922, 47th year, pp. 32-72 and pp. 235-258. This last study contains a complete critical summary, excellent from every point of view, of the psycho-physiological problem of the nature of emotion.

[2] There can, however, be no doubt that in the normal course of the activity of an organism the cortical functions intervene to ensure the complex realization of the instincts. Localized cortical disturbances may involve disturbances in the instinctive activities, if only through diachisis. But we cannot infer

An external stimulus which brings the tendencies into play not only provokes definite reactions and more or less appropriate reflexes, but also produces general manifestations of activity subject to a certain orientation.

The affective interest aroused by the stimulation is shown by a general liberation of nervous energy, partially canalized in certain preferential tracts. Unlike the reflex, a partial response of limited duration with a well-defined mechanism, the affective response involves a comparatively persistent total activity. And in the normal organism, a large part of this activity takes place in the association area. Mental functioning is powerfully aroused by the affective reaction which is registered, in connection with perceptions, images and ideas, in the form of a particular impression, sentiment or emotion, according to our psychological terminology.

But as a matter of fact, it seems that the character of 'emotion' belongs to affective impressions intense enough to involve an excessive liberation of nervous energy, which is no longer confined even to the reinforcement of the adapted reactions, but extends beyond the nervous reaction tracts, according to Lapicque,[1] and involves various manifestations of activity, not only in the form of motor agitation, as in exuberance of joy, but in the form of organic, visceral, secretory and other modifications. Excitor or inhibitory reactions are thus released, which accelerate or retard the heart, dilate or contract the peripheral vessels and so cause blushing or paleness, arrest gastric secretion, increase sweating, salivation and lachrymal secretion, cause intestinal contractions and colic, relax the sphincters, dilate the pupils, etc.

from this, as does Paulesco, on the basis of experiments by no means convincing, the cortical localization of the instincts (*cf.* N. C. Paulesco, "Localisation des instincts sur l'écorce cérébrale," *Archiv. intern. de Physiologie*, XIX, 1, 1922, pp. 74-87).

[1] L. Lapicque, "Essai d'une nouvelle théorie physiologique de l'emotion," *Journal de Psychologie*, 1911, VIII, pp. 1-8.

All these emotional reactions, for which childish explanations have been sought in terms of purpose, appear to be exaggerated consequences of the fundamental phenomenon of affectivity, the liberation of nervous energy;[1] they react in their turn by their coenæsthetic reverberation on the affective area, prolonging the emotional reaction; and they penetrate into the association area and contribute to form the mental complex registered in our experience as 'emotion,' with the specific characteristics of joy, fear, or anger, involving different orientations of the activity of the organism as a whole.

A peripheral excitation, such as a sweet perfume or a sudden burn, will arouse a response from the thalamo-striate[2] affective centre, which will be stronger in the absence of the cortical inhibition that normally influences all centres of immediate response, to the advantage of elaborated reactions. But with even more efficacy an associative representation or a perception, such as the hearing of good or bad news, a pleasant or an unpleasant sight, will arouse the affective mechanisms whose effects will be felt both on all the lower nervous centres and on the cortical area itself, on thought.

Were it reduced to the affective area, the organism would be deprived on the one hand of all the perceptive and representative sources of emotion, that is to say of almost all its sources in the case of man, and, on the other, of the immediate intellectual reverberations of the emotional reaction, as well as the indirect reverberations due to subsequent organic modifications; it would be deprived of the knowledge of the affective state,

[1] *Cf.* H. Piéron, "Les formes élémentaires de l'émotion dans le comportement animal. La dynamogénie émotionelle," *Journal de Psychologie*, 1920, XVII, pp. 937-945.

[2] According to Buscaino, the mesencephalon, as well as the thalamencephalon, forms part of the affective sphere: "Il cervello intermedio ed il mesencefalo," he says, "assumono quindi una importanza fondamentale nel meccanismo dei processi psichici. Essi costituiscono la zona alla cui funzione è dovuto se un fatto mentale assume o no una data tonalita emotiva" ("I centri encefalici dei reflessi emotivi," *Rivista di Psicologia*, 1920, 3-4).

that is to say, of its registration by experience, of its action on further behaviour: so that, instead of seeking in advance the means of favouring the agreeable impression, or of avoiding the renewal of the painful emotion, a purely affective organism would remain as before when confronted by analogous stimuli, able only to react in their presence in the same way and when actually touched off; for the emotion, as objectively characterized above, could not become a mental event[1] and so of service for a more perfect adaptation of activity and conduct.

The adaptation, which would thus be lacking, would consist in an action on events, and sometimes on the organism, in an effort to inhibit painful affective reactions, either when such events were inevitable, or when, as a result of sufficiently strong tendencies of social origin, they should not be avoided—for example, in the case of some danger faced in the spirit of social sacrifice.

[1] Is consciousness attached to the primary emotion, to the affective impression of the sub-cortical centres, directing the general reactions of the organism, or only to the mental registration, to the associative knowledge of the emotional reactions? This is a problem which it is useless to raise, since it is quite insoluble.

CHAPTER IV

THE DATA OF AFFECTIVE PATHOLOGY

THERE are isolated disturbances of the affective area: painful irritability with crises of agonized exasperation, such as we find in cases of causalgia, where the sympathetic fibres have aroused erethism in the centres at the base of the brain, or in most of the thalamic syndromes; the states of anger which are frequent in epileptics, though they may constitute isolated syndromes such as were observed in certain cases after war traumata, and which appear to be connected, in Huntington's chorea, with an injury to the basal ganglia; and those very common states of anxiety, 'anxiety neuroses,' which are attributed by Freudians to a conflict of sexual tendencies.

But in mental disorders affective pathology also plays a considerable part; and though long neglected in favour of intellectual disorders, it was rehabilitated by Pierre Janet and then glorified by Freud.

In dealing with the exaltation of maniacs and their incoherent agitation, we must not look for the mechanism of their disorders in the sphere of association. Pierre Janet sees here the effect of an excessive liberation of energy for the available psychic 'tension,' which involves agitation and waste in lower forms of activity, while, if the 'potential' of action were higher, an equal quantity of liberated activity would produce complex actions, at a high level of attention, and superior 'energy.'

It might also be held that in the case of excessive discharges, the mechanisms of inhibition which are necessary for the higher forms of mental functioning are overcome by too powerful excitations, in a dynamogenic form, characteristic of joy; and in fact, in the case of serious people, news productive of violent joy sometimes involves temporary agitation, with an incapacity to attend, and produces childish and incoherent actions, very like a minor maniacal attack.

Whatever may be the truth with regard to this important question of mechanism, it is certain that the origin of these disorders should be sought in the regulation of nervous activity and of the expenditure of energy, that is to say in the affective sphere.

True melancholia — in so far as it is not a mere depression due to diminution of activity, or to weariness after excessive expenditure, of which the repeated emotions of the war, which absorbed so much energy, provided countless examples—might appear to be a specific inverse injury, an excessive expenditure, directed especially into the tracts of inhibition and arrest, but also capable of appearing as an anxiety agitation.

In most of the obsessions, as already appears in Pierre Janet's penetrating analysis, which psychoanalysis with its systematic deformations has continued, the affective injury is at the root of the intellectual disorder.

And the analysis of many cases of madness leads us to make a disequilibration of tendencies the cause of those disorders of the reasoning faculties, so many examples of which are provided in normal cases by affective logic, in Ribot's sense (Rignano's "intentional reasoning").

Finally, it is the complete extinction of affectivity which, at any rate at the outset, seems alone to be in operation in certain forms of 'dementia precox'[1]

[1] Dide and Guiraud call dementia præcox an 'athymhormia,' or a loss of the *élan vital*, and regard it as an hereditary affection connected with the involution of the terminal cells of the sympathetic tracts controlling coenæsthesia and the direction of the instinctive vital activity located in the subthalamic region (*Psychiatrie du médecin practicien*, Paris, 1922).

where social life is rendered impossible through incoherence and complete lack of adaptation of conduct; and this mental impotence is often found where the associative functions are intact, and where only directive unity is lacking. We see here what can happen when a cortical function is no longer controlled by the area of the affective impressions that regulates the tendencies, when the automatisms are released without purpose and systematization, when absolute indifference reigns, and there is neither disgust,[1] nor shame, nor pain nor joy. The dementia seems more profound than when the intellectual mechanisms are lacking, and when tendencies regulating a certain biological and social activity still persist.

Governing the higher mental activity—which reacts upon it—the affective area, where the biological unity of the organism[2] is co-ordinated, is in close connection not only with the whole integrative nervous system, but also with the entire system of organic life. The reverberations of the sympathetic, including in this the 'parasympathetics,' make themselves felt with an extreme violence. And chemical actions, the secretory influences transmitted through the vascular tract, also exercise an organic direction of tendencies, and thereby of mental life as a whole.

Though certain toxic actions result in the excitation

[1] *Dementia præcox* patients, for example, will eat their excrement without disgust. Disgust may either be of intellectual origin or it may acquire an intellectual character in consequence of the coenæsthetic impressions that accompany a reflex nausea, through the introduction of certain nauseating substances into the stomach; in any case conduct is governed only by the affective impression of disgust. If this impression is lacking, the cortical mechanisms will not in all cases suffice, in spite of the acquired automatisms, to prevent certain acts and to promote others. Any association of ideas whatever will suffice to produce an absurd and disgusting activity, no longer inhibited by the affective brake.

[2] In his interesting general study, where he shows how the nervous system plays the rôle of intermediary between the exterior and the interior and between various parts of the body, van Rijnbeck recalls the fact that the unity of the living being is connected with the nervous system. But the unity of this unity is, in my opinion, to be found in the affective sphere (*cf.* van Rijnbeck "Rôle et organisation du système nerveux," *Arch. neerl. de Physiologie*, I, 1917, pp. 198-225).

of the cortical area, producing for example hallucinations of sight or touch, there are some which manifest a very active influence on affectivity, like adrenalin, which produces, in a sufficiently strong dose, a state of anxiety (Marañon), or chloride of β-tetrahydronaphthylamine, which produces in the cat all the symptoms of the most violent rage, even when the animal is 'apesthetized' (Elliott), or hyoscine, which suppresses sexual desire and certain essences which produce an impression of euphoria, etc.; and all these affective modifications quickly lead to intellectual justification.

Adrenalin, secreted by the supra-renals, is perhaps an agent of emotional reverberation; in any case, we know that hormones, produced by internal secretions poured into the circulation, act specifically to awaken or calm tendencies and thus to govern the conduct of an organism, and indirectly orientate all its intellectual activity.[1]

The genital hormones, at puberty, awaken the instincts, enliven the emotions, and involve liberations of energy, and so play an essential part in the mental life of the adolescent. In their absence, the principal centre of intellectual activity is extinguished: the æsthetic emotions are effaced, the disinterested tendencies grow weak and disappear. Social automatisms and acquired habits, still easy to release, may persist, but impulses are lacking.[2]

[1] We may further connect with these data the part played by a substance elaborated by the liver, which is necessary to the functioning of the nervous system and particularly of certain centres: thus an interruption of the hepatic circulation suppresses pain and allows operations on a dog without anæsthesia, whereas the introduction of blood from an animal with hepatic circulation produces algesic sensibility (Renauld-Capart, "Contribution a l'étude du metabolisme cérébral," *Arch. interm. de Physiologie*, XV, p. 244 and p. 411, XVI, p. 21 and p. 119).

[2] I have observed, as a consequence of serious and repeated emotional shocks, very curious cases of infantilism in adults, where complete amnesia, accompanying sexual inhibition and disturbances of the affective area, produced the mentality and conduct of a little child. In one case, social re-education, of an intellectual nature, was able to restore the acquired attitudes of the adult, but the infantile character persisted, together with sexual incapacity

Pézard has shown in the case of cocks the curious reversals which the ablation or grafting of the male or female genital glands can produce in character and behaviour, as well as in certain morphological characteristics.

We know that the ligature of the vas deferens in the case of old dogs or old rats suffices to give them a new vigour, a renewed nervous activity and the tendencies of youth: the indifference of the old animal gives place to susceptibility in the male, to care in the toilet, and to a desire for the chase (Steinach).

Then, too, there is the 'suprarenal virility' of girls affected with a tumour of the adrenals, resulting in a complete sexual inversion, psychical as well as physical, with all the masculine characteristics and tastes.

The maternal instinct, which has so great an influence on conduct and thought, is also governed by organic factors. Rabaud has demonstrated a development of maternal love in mice at a certain stage of pregnancy, under influences which are obviously humoral.[1]

These powerful organic actions enter the thalamo-striate affective area, in close connection with the vegetative life, and through this they exercise an influence on the neo-mental area, and on intellectual associations.

We shall, therefore, fail to understand the cortical mechanisms of thought if we consider them in isolation; they must be connected with motor apparatus of an organic nature; intelligence is an instrument of life which does not contain in itself the key to its own activity.

It is obviously vain to look for cortical lesions in most cases of insanity and in many forms of mental alienation, as if associative disorders were responsible, whereas essentially there is only a disturbance of the

(*cf.* H. Piéron "Le Puérilisme. Essai d'analyse du syndrome de Dupré à propos des puérils de guerre," *Revue de Médecine*, 1919, pp. 300-345, and pp. 410-437).

[1] E. Rabaud, "L'instinct maternal ches les mammifères," *Journal de Psychologie*, 1921, XVIII 6, pp. 487-495.

tendencies, an injury to the affective area, often itself secondary to an endocrine imbalance, that is to say to an affection belonging to general pathology.

Certainly our knowledge of the precise mechanisms through which the hormones modify the thalamo-striate centres, and through which the modification of these centres reverberates in changes of orientation of behaviour, in influences directing the play of cortical associations, the dynamic machinery of thought, is still insufficient and very rudimentary. Even the psychological analysis of the play of feelings and of their rôle in mental activity, so long neglected, is far from complete. Finally, the mechanism of social sublimation through collective influences, which are exercised on the fiercely egoistic biological tendencies of the organism, and results in human spirituality, has not yet been fully elucidated. To sum up, we can arrange the phenomena according to their main lines, and the progress of psycho-physiological knowledge in this respect is genuine; it is certainly calculated to encourage us in our further research.

CONCLUSION

In concluding this outline, if we cast a backward glance it seems that thanks to converging efforts, psychology and physiology are being linked together with positive and useful results.

Little by little we succeed in freeing ourselves from the congealed concepts of traditional psychology, which, up to the present, has rather sought to reconstruct man as he ought to be, in accordance with the exigencies of logic and morality, than to analyse him as a datum of fact, in accordance with the methods of the natural sciences. To-day we generally refuse to let ourselves be hypnotized by the insoluble problem of consciousness, and limit ourselves to the objective standpoint of the analysis of communicable, registrable facts, by which our social heritage may be enriched. We are engaged in constructing a science of psychology, dynamic in spirit, which forms an integral part of the biological sciences.

This psychology determines the laws of the general activity of organisms, in their relations with the environment. Thanks to the marvellous and delicate instrument of language, human psychology can study minute phenomena, and can penetrate into the details of an extraordinarily complex activity. Physiology, on the other hand, which addresses itself to the nervous mechanisms that produce the reactions observed by the psychologist, cannot reach the details. Its progress is, however, enormous, since the time when that pioneer Gall, who has been so unjustly misunderstood, imagined a fusion of psychology and cerebral physiology.[1]

The anatomical and morphological spirit, which can only conceive of convolutions or cell masses—corresponding to the static spirit of most of the psychologists of the last century, which was sustained by entities, images or concepts—has been the source of confusions and errors which have obscured the problem of cerebral localization.[2]

In order to understand the functioning of the brain, nervous functioning must first be understood;[3] and in this respect the labours of the French school of Lapicque are of fundamental importance. Though we have not as yet a completely satisfying explanation of the elementary nervous mechanisms, at least we are fairly sure of the main lines of this explanation. We know also that every nervous process represents the activation of a comparatively complex chain of neurones, often very far removed from one another, and that this chain,

[1] Phrenology seems childish to us to-day, but Gall was an innovator whose influence was considerable and fruitful, and Blondel has rightly attempted a rehabilitation. (*Cf. La Psychophysiologie de Gall*, Paris 1914).

In reality Gall, who lacked an anatomo-physiological basis and had not analysed the entities of the faculty-psychology, could never produce more than ridiculous schemata. Less pardonable are the imaginary schemata of a number of more recent authors, like Grasset's polygon and centre O, which, however, had a great success.

[2] The anatomists are always hoping to make psychological and morphological data directly correspond. Vogt, to whom we owe an admirable work on the architectonics of the cerebral cortex, thus concluded the lectures he gave in Paris in 1910: "By examining, during their lifetime, a certain number of individuals with the aid of these psychological methods and then studying the architecture of their brains, we may hope to find the anatomical characteristic of their intellectual qualities, and thus to advance the science of cerebral localization." In this attempt to establish a connection he neglects the essential link, which is physiological (*cf.* Oskar Vogt, "Quelques considérations générales sur la myélo-architecture du lobe frontal," *Revue Neurologique*, April 15, 1910, p. 420.)

[3] But certain naive followers of Watson, 'Behaviorists' of the American school, who take for their motto "Give me a nerve and a muscle and I will make you a mind," regard it as useless to penetrate into the 'cerebral mystery' to explain thought, which consists for them in neuro-muscular peripheral processes! *Cf.* Givler, *Journal of Philosophy*, 1921, XVIII, pp. 617-629.

since it undergoes many and various influences from other groups, cannot be isolated without a profound modification of function.

As there are many millions of these chains of neurones in the brain, we can realize how confused must be the modifications due to localized excitation or destruction, which, in the case of man, who alone can be studied in sufficient detail, thanks to language, are generally due only to the chance of blind natural experiments.

And yet, as we have seen, these blind experiments have yielded a rich harvest of facts. The truth is that in the chains of neurones constituting functional circuits of thought, there are systematic groups, connecting groups especially, which justify the idea of 'centres.' These centres are critical areas where mechanisms with a distinct rôle are articulated: receptive and incito-associative connections; projective and incito-motor connections; connections of co-ordination and elaboration, perceptive and executive. The value of the facts obtained is such that psychical symptoms admit of neurological diagnosis, the diagnosis of lesions in centres, and if required, can direct the surgeon's trepan.

On the other hand, the delicate mehods of histology support the findings of physiology, they describe the connecting elements, and follow the receptive and projective tracts and the great association paths; and, we can even, thanks to the degeneration produced by a lesion of groups of fibres, at any one point, distinguish the course of given bundles in the midst of thousands of others.

While a physiologist like Sherrington, and a psychologist like McDougall, have shown that the data furnished by each retina, fused into binocular perception, really enjoy a relative automony in spite of powerful unifying associations, an anatomist like Minkowski has concurrently proved that the connecting tracts of each retina retain their individuality and their independence as far as the calcarine cortex, where they both come to an end in the area of visual reception that contains powerful association paths (bundle of Vicq-d'Azyr) found nowhere else.

Moreover physiology forms an efficient supplement to psychological analysis by providing evidence along its own lines of phenomena identical with those otherwise made known to us by the study of the mind.[1] When Graham Brown shows that the preliminary excitation of a point on the cortex facilitates the excitation of adjacent points or the immediately consecutive excitation of the same point, he is concerned with the very phenomenon with which we are already familiar—the lowering of the threshold of sensation by a preliminary or simultaneously associated excitation and which we call involuntary attention. The reinforcements and inhibitions which constitute attention are very general data of neuro-physiology.

By his method of the conditioned reflex which has proved so fruitful, Pavlov has succeeded in advancing from the physiological point of view questions which seemed to belong essentially to the psychological domain: attention, memory, the law of association, and sensory analysis. But he regards psychology, with a terminology full of subjective significations, as useless if not harmful, since he cannot conceive the possibility of an objective attitude in mental analysis, which he thinks is merely an effort at explanation in terms of consciousness, thus showing himself somewhat ill-informed.

We may certainly admit that very valuable data as to the fundamental laws of the special activity of the cortex, an 'analysing' activity, are furnished by the method of the conditioned reflex, a method which does not involve the direct isolation of the cerebral tracts activated, and has much in common with the methods of training employed in animal psychology. But it

[1] *Cf.* Geo. T. Johnson, "A Survey of the Physiology of Cerebration," *Journal of Abn. Psychology*, 1921, XVI, pp. 115-136.

is none the less true that this activity of the cortex, whose delicacy and precise gradation Head, from his point of view, rightly emphasizes, can be followed in its complexity only by means of the social instrument constituted by language with its nice gradations, especially the very rich languages bequeathed to us by the great European civilizations.

The fundamental laws may perhaps then appear less clearly than in a general study,[1] but if these laws are presupposed, we can better follow their forms and variations in the rich domain of verbal reactions where human psychology displays all its powers of analysis.

Thus the knowledge of human mental functions—so invaluable for us—will continue to progress on the foundations of the neuro-physiology and histomorphology of the brain. It will profit by the evolutionary data of animal psychology, and will utilize the sociological discoveries which retrace the special laws of collective influences or follow the acquisition of instruments of thought transmitted to new generations; and above all, it will be derived from the direct investigation of human behaviour.

[1] Thus, by following his own method, Pavlov has established a very general law, that of "irradiation and subsequent concentration of the nervous process," and he shows that the psychological approach would not admit of a general representation of this law. (*Cf.* J. P. Pavlov, "La vraie physiologie cérébrale," *Archives internat. de Physiol.* 1921, XVIII, pp. 607-616. This study represents a communication to the Congress of Psychiatry, Neurology and Psychology which should have taken place in August 1914.)

INDEX

For Product Safety Concerns and Information please contact our EU representative GPSR@taylorandfrancis.com
Taylor & Francis Verlag GmbH, Kaufingerstraße 24, 80331 München, Germany

www.ingramcontent.com/pod-product-compliance
Lightning Source LLC
LaVergne TN
LVHW011119300926
849160LV00008B/444